# PRACTICAL GUIDE TO RESPIRATOR USAGE IN INDUSTRY

# PRACTICAL GUIDE TO RESPIRATOR USAGE IN INDUSTRY

*Gyan S. Rajhans*
*David S.L. Blackwell*

**BUTTERWORTH PUBLISHERS**
Boston · London
Sydney · Wellington · Durban · Toronto

**Library of Congress Cataloging in Publication Data**

Rajhans, Gyan S.
Practical guide to respirator usage in industry.

   Includes index.
   1. Respirators.  2. Respiratory organs—Diseases—
Prevention.  3. Gases, Asphyxiating and poisonous—Safety
measures.  4. Industrial safety—Equipment and supplies.
I. Blackwell, David S. L.  II. Title.
T55.3.G3R35  1985        602'.8'9         85–5734
ISBN 0–250–40477–X

Butterworth Publishers
80 Montvale Avenue
Stoneham, MA 02180

10 9 8 7 6 5 4 3 2 1

*Printed in the United States of America*

# Contents

# The Authors

Mr. Rajhans received a B.Sc. Eng. from Ranchi University at Bihar, India in 1963 and a M.Sc. in Engineering from Queen's University at Kingston, Ontario in 1966. In 1968 he was appointed Dust Control Specialist for the Occupational Health Engineering Service of the Ontario Ministry of Labour and in 1977 was promoted to Chief of this service. Mr. Rajhans is a registered Professional Engineer in Ontario; he is certified as a Specialist in Occupational Health Engineering by the Association of Professional Engineers of Ontario and is a C.I.H. in Engineering Aspects. Since 1972 he has been a member of both the Air Sampling Instruments and Industrial Ventilation Committees of ACGIH. He is also a member of the Editorial Board of AIHA *Journal*. Mr. Rajhans is the coauthor of *Engineering Aspects of Asbestos Dust Control* and *Asbestos Sampling and Analysis*.

Dr. Blackwell received a B.Sc. in Chemistry in 1970 and a Ph.D. in Organic Photochemistry in 1975 from the University of Western Ontario. He expanded his work from analytical chemistry to industrial hygiene and in 1978 became Supervisor of Industrial Hygiene/Analytical Chemistry at 3M Canada. He became Supervisor of the Occupational Health & Safety Products Laboratory at 3M in 1981 and is now Technical Manager of the Traffic & Personal Safety Products Division. Dr. Blackwell is a member of the American Industrial Hygiene Association and has held executive positions in the Occupational Hygiene Association of Ontario. He is a member of the Canadian Standard Association Technical Committee on Selection, Care and Use of Respirators, and is an associate member of the Canadian Standards Association Advisory Committee on Occupational Health and Safety Products.

# Preface

We live in an industrial world. Since man's first appearance on earth he has been a curious animal. From the fatal bite of the apple in the Garden of Eden through today and beyond, man has been and continues to be interested in the world around him, why things happen, what is new, how he can better his life, etc. This curiosity is responsible for the lifestyle we enjoy today and would not be willing to give up. What would we do without the technologies that exist today and those that are on the brink of being discovered? We have discovered thousands and thousands of chemicals which have enabled us to live the way we do. What would we do without plastics, polymers, pesticides, and drugs, just to name a few? Although most, if not all, of these chemicals are beneficial to the human race, many employees involved in their manufacturing, processing, handling, storage, etc., may be exposed to unhealthy levels of toxic materials in the workplace.

In the 1970s public awareness and concern about the effects of hazardous substances increased dramatically. The Assistant Surgeon General of the United States estimated that half a million chemicals were being produced and used in the United States and that approximately three thousand new chemicals were being developed annually. During the 1970s most industrialized nations produced at least one major report or study focusing on these heightened concerns. The Ham Commission in Ontario, the Rohens Report in the United Kingdom, and the Williams and Steiger Occupational Safety and Health Act in the United States are but three examples. A clear consensus on the growing threat to health from chemicals and other substances emerged, as well as the decision that it was necessary to control these hazards and that more comprehensive legislative measures were necessary.

Most occupational health and safety legislation promulgated in industrialized nations has placed the responsibility for a safe and healthy workplace on the employer, and he must accomplish this through the use of engineering control methods. Where these methods to control the workplace environment do not exist or are unavailable, i.e., are not reasonable or practical for the length of time or frequency of exposure, or the nature of the operation, process or work, or are not effective because of a temporary breakdown of equipment; personal protective equipment is used to provide necessary protection.

According to the *Concise Oxford Dictionary,* a respirator is defined as an "apparatus worn over mouth and nose to warm or filter inhaled air or to prevent inhalation of poison gas." The use of respiratory protection to filter out dusts, gases, vapors, mists and fumes from the air is not new. As early as A.D. 50 there is reference to the use of animal bladders by Romans to protect against the inhalation of red oxide of lead. During the time between the 1400s and the 1700s people like Leonardo da Vinci (1452–1519) and Bernardino Ramazzini (1633–1714) saw the need for respiratory protection against hazardous materials.

During the industrial revolution (1800s) respiratory protection progressed with contributions such as a "smoke filter" for firemen (1825) developed by John Roberts. It was in 1814 that the precursor to the modern day air-purifying respirator was developed. The most rapid period of evolution in design and function of respirators occurred during World War I when toxic war gases were first used as a military weapon. Since then respirators have been developed to provide adequate protection for almost every kind of work situation.

The development of respiratory protection continues today and will continue into the future. We do not have the perfect system. Chapter 9 discusses future research that is required in the field of respiratory protection. This work is not only needed on the respirator itself, but also on the respirator-person interface with emphasis on the person component.

Inhalation is the major route of entry of toxic materials into the human body. As mentioned earlier, respiratory protection is permitted where, for whatever reason, engineering controls fail to provide adequate protection. This book is a guide for the employer and employee who use respiratory protection, and it is not an attempt to give a detailed look at all the published literature on respiratory protection. It provides a guide to the plant manager, safety officer, plant nurse, industrial hygienist, etc., who have to develop and implement a complete respiratory protection program.

In order to comply with the Occupational Safety and Health Administration's Respiratory Protection Standard 1910.134 and to provide the necessary protection to employees, a respiratory protection program with the following minimum requirements is needed:

1. Written operating procedures outlining the entire program;
2. Procedures for proper selection of respirators;
3. Procedures for training users in the proper use and limitations of respirators;
4. Cleaning, maintenance, and storage procedures;
5. Inspection;
6. Medical surveillance of respirator users.

This book details the total respiratory protection program and each of its individual components. There are a large number of different types of respirators available to select from and the selection procedure can be complex. It is not enough to select the appropriate respirator, give it to the worker and assume that he is protected. Proper fitting, training, maintenance, inspection and storage are required. Also, it is necessary to be aware of what legal responsibilities are involved in respirator use.

It is our hope that this book will aid the user in the establishment of a proper respiratory protection program which will protect the health of his workers.

The authors gratefully acknowledge the contribution of June Rae and Kathie Anderson whose diligent typing made this book possible. Appreciation is also extended to Yolanda Hambridge whose proofreading and comments were invaluable.

*G.S.R.*
*D.S.L.B.*

# 1

# *Overview of Respiratory Hazards and Evaluation*

The type and extent of respiratory hazards present in the modern industrial environment dictates the selection of proper respirators. As several good texts are available on this subject, we will give only an overview of respiratory hazards encountered in industrial workplaces, and the various methods of evaluating them.

The main categories of hazards are shown in Figure 1.1. In the case of respirators, we are mainly concerned with chemical hazards.

Any chemical that has the capacity to produce injury or illness when taken into the body is called a toxic agent. In order that an agent develop toxic activities, it has to enter the body, be distributed to the body, and react with components of the body.

The human body has the capacity to get rid of ingested or inhaled noxious agents by vomiting, coughing and excretion. Healthy skin, for example, will not absorb water-soluble substances, therefore only substances which dissolve in body fluids can prove to be toxic. Lead sulfide, for example, cannot be dissolved either in water or in body fluids, and is therefore not toxic, whereas other lead compounds, which can be dissolved, will have a toxic action on the body. Another example is the iron compounds. Taken in large amounts they are toxic, however, since they are corrosive and locally irritating in the stomach they will be expelled from the stomach by vomiting before they can be absorbed.

To sum up, in order to become toxic, an agent must be absorbed into the body, be dissolved in body fluids, and interfere with metabolism.

For example, all lead compounds are inherently toxic; however, lead sulfide will not dissolve in body fluids unless taken by mouth. It is then transformed into lead chloride by hydrochloric acid in stomach juices. This is why its toxicity under industrial conditions is low.

On the other hand, a hazardous chemical can be defined as carrying with it the high probability that its use will cause biological effects in the body. Any given chemical agent may have intrinsic toxicity, but it may not

1

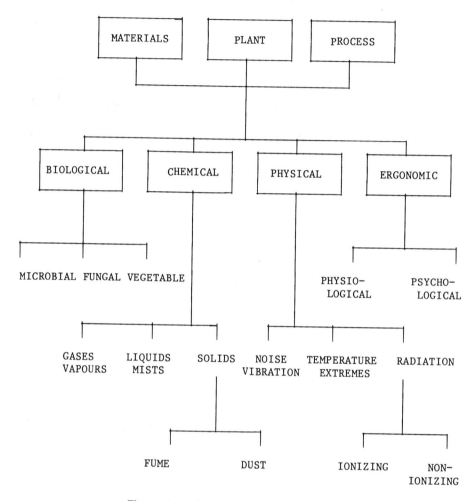

**Figure 1.1**  Occupational health hazards.

actually represent a health hazard unless the amount or the concentration that enters the body is sufficient to cause injury.

An example is trichloroethylene and perchloroethylene. Both are chlorinated hydrocarbons widely used in industry as solvents. Both produce the same toxic symptoms; however, the vapor pressure of trichloroethylene is 70 mm. Hg at 25°C, whereas the vapor pressure of perchloroethylene is only 23 mm. Hg at 25°C. This means that at the same room temperature much more trichloroethylene will evaporate and its concentration in the inhaled air will be much higher than the concentration of perchloroethylene vapors would be. The toxicity of both compounds is the same; however, the hazard associated with perchloroethylene is lower since the concentration of its vapor in the inhaled air will be, under equal conditions, much lower.

## ENTRY ROUTES FOR TOXIC SUBSTANCES

There are three ways in which chemical agents can enter the body:

1. By inhalation through the respiratory tract,
2. By ingestion into the digestive tract by eating or swallowing, and
3. By contact with, or absorption through, the skin.

As far as the use of respirators is concerned, the most important route of entry is by inhalation. Hence, the mechanism of inhalation is discussed in detail.

The lungs have an extremely large surface area (approximately 140 square meters including the alveolar surface and the blood capillary network surface) which provides a contact for the toxic materials. The large volume of air that is taken into the lungs on a daily basis, and the rapid rate of absorption from the air in the alveoli into the blood stream, make the respiratory tract the primary route for toxic materials to enter the body.

The primary function of the respiratory system is to provide a means for the exchange of oxygen and carbon dioxide (Fig. 1.2). Inhaled air enters the respiratory tract and is transported to the alveoli of the lungs. The alveoli are in close contact with blood capillaries and, because of concentration differences, oxygen diffuses from the alveoli to blood and the carbon dioxide diffuses from blood in the capillaries to the alveoli. Once oxygen reaches blood it combines with hemoglobin in the blood and is transported through the blood stream to the cells. In the cells oxygen is released from blood to provide food, which is necessary for cell life. In return, cells produce carbon dioxide as a waste by-product. This carbon dioxide is released into the blood stream and transported back to the lungs where it diffuses into the lungs and is exhaled out of the body. The large surface area and the minute separation between the alveoli and the capillary system make the lungs an efficient organ for the absorption of toxicants. These toxicants can be in the form of gases, solids or liquid aerosols. Many toxicants are capable of being transported from the lungs to other parts of the body and exerting their toxic effects. Toxicants which exert direct action on the lungs can, and do, cause effects on the gas exchange process which can have acute and/or chronic effects on one's health.

The lungs are also involved in the excretion of toxicants which have entered the body through the skin or have been ingested. Clearance of toxicants that reach the respiratory system is vitally important to proper respiratory function. Breakdown of these clearance mechanisms can have adverse effects on one's health.

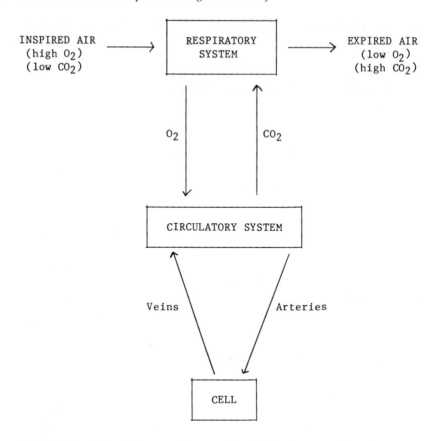

**Figure 1.2**  Role of the respiratory system in the transportation of oxygen and carbon dioxide.

## STRUCTURE OF THE RESPIRATORY TRACT

The respiratory tract consists of three major areas: the nasopharyngeal; the tracheobronchial; and the pulmonary (see Figure 1.3).

The nasopharyngeal area consists of the nose, pharynx and the larynx. The nose consists of an external portion which is mainly bone, cartilage and tissue, and an internal portion. This internal portion is composed of two wedge shaped cavities separated by a septum. The internal portion is covered by a thick mucous membrane which functions to warm and moisten inhaled air. The nose filters in two ways. The hairs that can be seen in the nose filter out the coarsest of foreign materials. The second filtration mode is via air currents passing over the moist mucous membranes in curved pathways and depositing fine particles against the wall. The trapped particles are subsequently carried to the pharynx and swallowed.

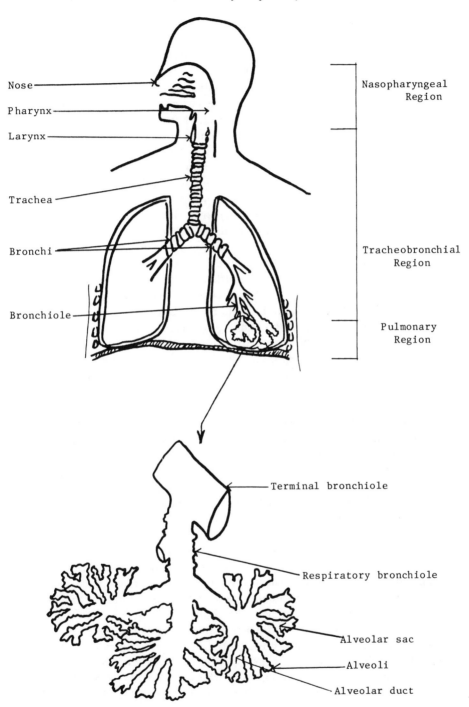

**Figure 1.3**   Schematic representation of the respiratory tract.

The pharynx is a musculomembranous tube, 5 inches in length, extending from the base of the skull to the esophagus. The pharynx is divided into three parts—nasal, oral and laryngeal. The pharynx serves as a passage for two systems—the respiratory and digestive systems.

The larynx, or voice box, connects the pharynx with the trachea. Its opening is at the base of the tongue. The larynx consists of nine cartilages united by muscles and ligaments. The chief function of the larynx is to vocalize. The pitch of the sound is determined by the shape and tension of the vocal cords. The voice is refined by the nose, mouth and pharynx, as well as the sinuses which act as sounding boards and resonating chambers.

Respiration starts when air is inhaled through the nose. The main function of the nasopharynx is to warm and moisten air and to filter and remove the largest particles ($> 10$ μm) from the air inhaled. The surfaces of the nose, sinus and the upper bronchi are covered with mucous membranes. These membranes secrete a fluid called mucus which is produced continuously and drains slowly into the throat. The mucus provides heat and humidity to the air chambers and thus warms incoming air. In addition to mucus, the membrane is coated with cilia (hairlike filaments) which wave back and forth. Millions of cilia line the nasopharyngeal area and aid in the cleaning of incoming air and the removal of deposited materials.

The tracheobronchial area consists of the trachea, bronchi and bronchiole. The trachea, or windpipe, is a cylindrical tube about 4 to 5 inches in length, consisting of cartilage separated by fibrous and muscular tissue. The trachea functions as a simple passageway for air passing to the lungs.

The bronchi consist of two separate passages which split off at the base of the trachea. The right bronchus differs from the left in that it is shorter and wider and takes a more vertical course. Because of this, foreign material tends to follow the right bronchus more often than the left. The bronchi become narrower as they approach the lungs. With this narrowing, the cartilage of the bronchi tends to be reduced and disappears at the bronchiole. The epithelial lining of the trachea loses its cilia and decreases in size.

The respiratory bronchiole are tubular with lengths of approximately 0.5 inches. There are many bronchiole branching off the bronchi. The walls are void of cartilage and contain only limited cilia.

The tracheobronchial areas serve as conducting airways between the nasopharynx and the alveoli where the gas exchange takes place. As in the nasopharynx, the tracheobronchial passageways are lined with cilia and coated with a thin layer of mucus. Medium-sized particles (1-10 μm) are filtered out in this region of the respiratory tract. The surface of these airways serves as a mucociliary escalator, moving particles from the deep lung to the oral cavities so that they can be swallowed or excreted.

The pulmonary section consists of the alveolar duct, the alveolar sac and the alveolus. It is here that gas exchange takes place between alveoli and blood capillaries. Particles less than 1 μm in size are deposited in this area. A more detailed description of the respiratory system can be found in the National Safety Council's book entitled *Fundamentals of Industrial Hygiene* [1].

Figure 1.4 illustrates volumes in respiration and represents the normal respiratory pattern at rest. Changes in volume and flow are recorded using a spirometer which is used to determine impairment to the respiratory system. The four primary lung volumes are:

1.  *Tidal Volume (TV).* The volume of gas inspired or expired during each respiratory cycle. Normally only a small volume of the lung is ventilated. The tidal volume is normally 500 ml.
2.  *Inspiratory Reserve Volume (IRV).* The maximum volume that can be forcibly expired following a normal inspiration. Typically this is 3300 ml. for men.

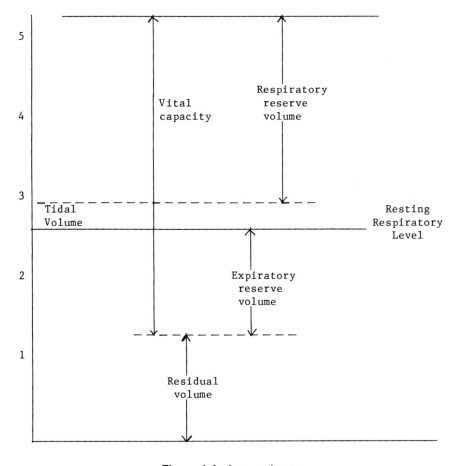

**Figure 1.4**   Lung volumes.

3. *Expiratory Reserve Volume (ERV)*. The maximum amount of air that can be forcibly expired following normal expiration. For men this is normally 1000 ml.
4. *Residual Volume (RV)*. The amount of air remaining in the lungs following a maximum expiratory effort. (Typically 1200 ml.).

Other volumes which are comprised of several of the primary ones are:

1. *Total Lung Capacity (TLC)*. The sum of all four volumes listed above.
2. *Inspiratory Capacity (IC)*. The maximum volume of air that can be inspired at the end of a normal tidal expiration (3800 ml. is average for men) (IC = IRV + TV)
3. *Vital Capacity (VC)*. The maximum amount of air that can be exhaled from the lungs following a maximum inspiration. (VC = IRV + TV + ERV) (4800 ml. is typical for a man).
4. *Functional Residual Capacity (FRC)*. The normal volume at the end of passive exhalation, that is, the gas volume which normally remains in the lung and functions as the residual capacity.

The flow of air from the lungs can be used as a tool in diagnosing changes in the lung. If the subject inhales and exhales maximally, the forced vital capacity (FVC) and forced expiratory volume at one second ($FEV_{1.0}$) can be recorded. The FVC is the maximal volume of air which can be exhaled forcefully after a maximal inspiration. The $FEV_{1.0}$ is that volume of air which can be forcibly expelled during the first second of expiration. Inhalation of toxicants may change the ability of the lungs to move air in and out due to obstruction or restriction of air passages. FVC and $FEV_{1.0}$ measurements can be used to detect these obstructions or restrictions in the lungs.

Factors which can cause changes in respiration include the partial pressure of carbon dioxide, the partial pressure of oxygen and the pH of arterial blood. Increased partial pressure of carbon dioxide in arterial blood increases respiration, while decreased partial pressure of carbon dioxide decreases respiration rate. On the other hand, decreased partial pressure of oxygen in arterial blood decreases respiration. A low arterial pH increases respiration rate. Pain, sudden cold and other sensory stimuli can elicit respiratory changes. Age is another factor influencing respiration rate. At birth the rate is rapid (from 40-70 times/minute). This rate decreases with age, so that at 1 year it is 35-40 times/minute; at 10 years, 20 times/minute; at 25 years, 16-18 times/minute. With old age, the rate can increase again to more than 20 times/minute. Body temperature affects the rate of respiration; increased body heat increases respiration.

## ACTION OF TOXICANTS IN THE RESPIRATORY SYSTEM

Once the toxic material has been inhaled its site of action and effect depend on a number of factors: chemical composition, chemical state, solubility, reactivity, etc. Inhaled contaminants that adversely affect the lungs fall into three major categories:

1. Aerosols/dusts which produce either tissue damage, tissue reaction, disease or physical plugging at the site of deposition.
2. Toxic gases that produce adverse reaction in the tissue of the lungs.
3. Toxic gases or aerosols that do not affect the lungs, but pass through the lungs and are transported, via the bloodstream, to other body organs.

### Gases and Vapors

Toxic gases and vapors may be inhaled and distributed throughout the entire respiratory system. While the exchange of oxygen and carbon dioxide can only take place deep in the lungs at the alveoli, intake of toxic gases and vapors can take place anywhere in the respiratory tract.

The diffusion of these toxic materials is the driving force behind the interaction of these gases and vapors within different regions of the respiratory tract. Usually there is a very small concentration of the toxicant in the tissues while there are higher concentrations in the inspired air. Diffusion is the phenomenon of a material moving from a high concentration to a low concentration. Thus it is the concentration differential which allows toxic gases and vapors to move from air to the tissues of the respiratory tract. The solubility of these toxic materials in water greatly influences the relative toxicity and the site of reaction in the respiratory tract. Very soluble gases, such as ammonia or sulfur dioxide are absorbed in the nasopharyngeal area, other gases such as nitrogen dioxide and organic solvent vapors are less soluble in water. They do not readily dissolve in the mucous membrane and are able to reach lower into the airways and can even reach the alveolar area, resulting in their diffusion into the bloodstream. In this latter category of toxicant the direct effect may not be on the lungs, rather their diffusion into the bloodstream may mean that other organs will be affected. Those toxicants that are very water-soluble react with the mucous layer of the respiratory tract. Since the mucous layer is always being renewed and removed by ingestion or carried to the mouth by the cilia, dissolution in this layer detoxifies the gas or vapor.

The lining of the upper portion of the respiratory tract is composed of mainly goblet and ciliated cells. The goblet cells are responsible for the secretion of mucus. If the toxic gas or vapor is capable of interfering with the goblet cells, then the rate of mucous secretion is affected. Once the toxicant has penetrated the mucous lining of the upper airways (highly water-soluble materials), the goblet and ciliated cells can be attacked. It appears that ciliated cells are more prone to the effects of toxic gases and vapors. Cilia may be lost and their cells may even die. This results in a lack of cilia in the area and the process which involves the removal of foreign materials can be greatly affected.

If the toxic gas or vapor is not very soluble in water, it will most likely reach the lower airways (alveoli) of the lungs. Once this occurs, the intake of the gas or vapor is the same as that for oxygen. That is, diffusion determines the fate of the toxicant. The alveoli are separated from the blood stream by a very thin lining and there are usually lower concentrations of the toxicant in the blood than in the alveoli; thus, via diffusion, gases and vapors are capable of moving into the blood stream. Even though toxic gases or vapors reach the lower airways, it does not mean that they will pass into the blood and not have toxic effects on the lower portion of the respiratory tract. Certain regions of the lower airway are more affected by gases and vapors that act directly on the lung. For example, ozone affects the region between the bronchiole and the alveolus more so than other areas of the body.

The respiratory system may also be exposed to toxic gases and vapors through its function in the excretory process. Vapors from organic compounds, such as benzene and toluene, are excreted through the lungs. If the metabolism of these vapors to more water-soluble metabolites is slow, high levels of vapors may be exhaled. Toxic materials absorbed by other routes, or toxic metabolites from other areas in the body, may be excreted through the respiratory system. The toxicants may then accumulate in a high concentration in the lungs, resulting in pulmonary damage.

## Particulate Material

Inhaled particulates can take many forms, commonly called "aerosols." An aerosol is a suspension of solid particles or liquid droplets in a gaseous medium. There are at least six forms of particulate materials which we must be concerned with:

1. *Dust.* Solid particles usually larger than colloid and capable of temporary suspensions in air or other gases which generally result from the application of physical force to a larger mass such as grinding, sanding, cutting, et cetera.
2. *Fog.* Visible aerosols in which the dispersed phase is liquid.
3. *Fume.* Solid particles generated by condensation from the gaseous state.
4. *Mist.* Dispersion of liquid particles.

5.  *Smog.* Atmospheric contamination by aerosols arising from a combination of natural and man-made sources.
6.  *Smoke.* Particles resulting from incomplete combustion.

The site of deposition in the respiratory tract plays a major role in the toxic effect of the inhaled aerosol. There are a number of factors which determine the site of deposition of the aerosol, namely size, density, shape, tendency to aggregate, etc. Particle size plays the major role in determining where the aerosol will settle out in the respiratory tract. Usually the inhaled particles are not uniform in size and shape. For simplicity, we consider all particles to be spheres of unit density and the size distribution of the aerosol approximates a lognormal distribution. We usually refer to the particle-size of the aerosol as the median or geometric mean particle-size. Also reference is usually made to the aerodynamic diameter of a particle which takes into account the density of the particle and the aerodynamic drag. The aerodynamic diameter represents the diameter of a unit density sphere having the same terminal settling velocity as the particle, whatever its size, shape and density. Aerosols can range in size from 0.01 μm to 100 μm. Figure 1.5 illustrates the type of aerosols and their typical particle size.

There are four mechanisms which influence the deposition of particulate material in the respiratory tract; these are interception, impaction, sedimentation and diffusion.

Interception occurs when the movement of the particle in the airways brings it into close proximity with the surface of the respiratory tract. By being in close proximity to the surface the particle is able to come into contact with the surface and is removed from the airstream. Interception plays a major role in particle filtering in the upper nasopharyngeal region and affects particles that are greater than 30 μm in size.

Impaction occurs when the airways make abrupt changes in direction as in the lower nasopharyngeal region. As the airways change direction, by momentum, the particle is forced to move in one direction and thus runs into the surface of the passageway. Particles in the 5-30 μm size range are strongly influenced by impaction and filtered out in the lower nasopharyngeal region. Airflow in the nasopharyngeal region is very high (> 180 cm./ sec.). This high airflow, and the tortuous nature of the air passages in this region, causes the airflow to change direction often. This provides the ideal condition for impaction to take place.

Sedimentation brings about the deposition of particles of the 1-5 μm size into the smaller bronchi and the bronchioles where the velocity of the airflow is low. As the particles move down the airways, buoyancy and resistance of air act on the particles in an upward direction while the gravitational forces act in a downward direction. Since the velocity of the air becomes less as it moves deeper into the lungs, the gravitational forces equal or exceed the sum of the buoyancy and air resistance. This results in the particles settling out on the surface of the bronchi and bronchioles.

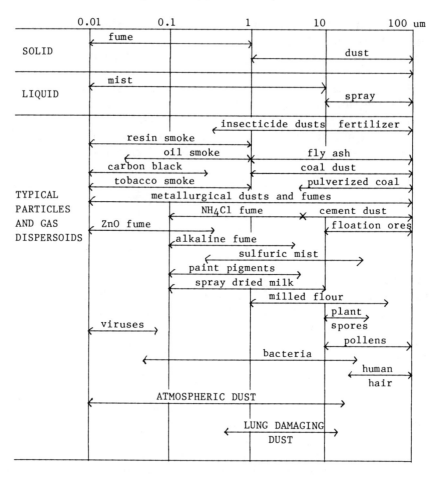

**Figure 1.5**   Sizes of airborne particles.

Diffusion is important in the aveolar region. Since the velocity of airflow in this region is very low, the particles begin to collide with gas molecules. Random motion is important to the particles in this process which is referred to as Brownian Motion. Brownian Motion increases with decreasing particle size, and its random motion causes the particles to come into contact with the aveoli surface and become deposited there. Particles of less then 1µm size distribution are affected by diffusion. Table 1.1 illustrates the complexity of the air passage, relative size and air velocity as the air goes from the trachea to the alveolar sacs. Table 1.2 summarizes the particle size of material filtered out in each region of the respiratory tract.

Breathing patterns influence particle deposition. During quiet breathing, in which the tidal volume is only two or three times the volume of the dead space, a large proportion of the inhaled particles may be exhaled.

Table 1.1   Components of the respiratory tract showing the complexity and air velocity in each region

| | | Number | X-Section (cm2) | Air Velocity cm/sec |
|---|---|---|---|---|
| **AIR CONDUCTION** | Air Conduction | | | |
| | Trachea | 1 | 1.3 | 150 |
| | Main Bronchi | 2 | 1.1 | 180 |
| | Primary and Segmental Bronchi | 880 | 1.5–14 | 130–14 |
| | Terminal Bronchioles | $5.4 \times 10^4$ | 150 | 1.3 |
| **GAS EXCHANGE** | Gas Exchange | | | |
| | Respiratory Bronchioles | $1.1 \times 10^5$ | 220 | 0.9 |
| | Alveolar Ducts | $2.6 \times 10^7$ | 820 | 0.025 |
| | Alveolar Sacs | $5.2 \times 10^7$ | $1.4 \times 105$ | 0 |

During exercise or heavy work larger volumes of air are inhaled at higher velocities; thus, the deposition mechanisms increase. Holding one's breath can also increase deposition by sedimentation and diffusion. Any constriction in the airways caused by irritant materials, sickness, diseases, etc., will increase the amount of particle deposition by impaction.

Table 1.2   Summary of deposition mechanism and particle size filtered in each region of the respiratory tract

| Respiratory Tract Region | Particle Size Filtered ($\mu$m) | Deposition Mechanism | Airflow Directional Changes | Air Velocity (cm/sec) |
|---|---|---|---|---|
| Upper Nasopharyngeal | > 30 | Interception | extremely abrupt | > 180 |
| Lower Nasopharyngeal | 5 – 30 | Impaction | very abrupt | > 180 |
| Tracheo-bronchial | 1 – 5 | Sedimentation | less abrupt | 1 – 130 |
| Pulmonary | < 1 | Diffusion | mild | 0 – 1 |

The respiratory tract has the capability of removing deposited particulate material from the site of deposition. This clearance mechanism varies depending on the site of deposition. In the nasopharyngeal and tracheobronchial regions the air passages are coated with cilia which are moving back and forth at all times. The particles trapped in the mucous coating of those regions are transported by a mucociliary escalator up to the mouth and are ingested.

Particulate material that is deposited in the alveolar region is subjected to three main avenues of clearance:

1.  Particles being phagocytized and cleared via the mucociliary escalator up the tracheobronchial tree,
2.  Particles being phagocytized and removed via lymphatic drainage, and
3.  Partial or complete dissolving of the particle and removal via the bloodstream or lymphatic drainage.

Within the alveolar region there is a large number of macrophages which engulf all particles within several hours of inhalation. The phagocytized particle is then capable of being cleared from the system via one of the three mechanisms listed above. Figure 1.6 summarizes the fate and effects of particulate material which has been inhaled.

In order for a toxic effect to occur in the human body, it is necessary for the toxicant to reach the appropriate site of action in a high enough concentration and to stay there long enough to exert its toxic effect. Thus, changes in dose, route and duration of exposure can influence the toxic effect. We will not be attempting to give a detailed summary of toxicology in this book, but we think that the reader should be aware of the variables (factors) which may influence the toxic effect of foreign material in the human body.

Factors which influence the toxicity of a material can be related to the toxic agent, the exposure, and the subject. These factors can be further divided. Table 1.3 summarizes the variables which can affect the toxicity of materials that enter the body.

In summary, the respiratory system is vulnerable to airborne contaminants. Depending on the nature of the inhaled material, the site of deposition, etc., certain toxic effects may be felt in the respiratory system itself (Table 1.4 summarizes some of these effects), or elsewhere in the body. The respiratory tract is an effective filtering system and is capable of removing the contaminant from the body. Irritation of the air passages resulting in constriction of the airways; damage to the cells lining the airways; production of fibrosis; constriction of the airways caused by allergic reactions; and production of lung tumors are the five general toxic responses of the respiratory system to airborne contaminants.

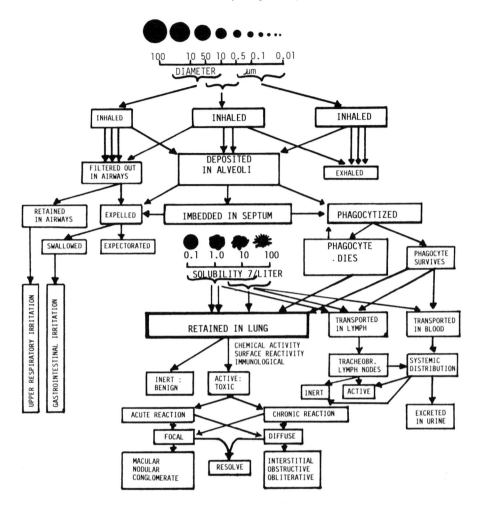

**Figure 1.6** Schematic presentation of the biological fate and effects of inhaled inorganic particulates (from *Archives of Environmental Health,* 1963).

## SOURCES OF RESPIRATORY HAZARDS

The wide variety of processes used in industry give rise to numerous potential health problems. In this chapter, for readers' ready use, we list examples of chemical substances associated with industrial processes (Table 1.5). The list is by no means complete either for processes or chemical contaminants, and is intended only as a guide.

The terms used in this table have been defined earlier in this chapter, however, they are described again below for easy reference.

Table 1.3   Summary of factors that influence the toxicity of materials entering the human body

---

```
1.  Factors related to the agent

            - Chemical composition
            - Physical composition
            - Solubility in biologic fluids
            - Presence of other materials


2.  Factors related to the exposure

            - Dose
            - Route of entry
            - Duration and frequency


3.  Factors related to the subject

            - Age, sex, body weight
            - Health status
            - Nutritional status
            - Genetic status
            - Environmental factors such as temperature,
              humidity, social factors, geographic influences,
              etc.
```

---

1.  *Dust.* Finely divided solid particles dispersed in air, which have been generated by mechanical processes such as grinding, crushing, blasting and drilling.
2.  *Fume.* Solid particles dispersed in air formed by the condensation of vapors of solid materials.
3.  *Gas.* An aeriform which does not become liquid or solid at ordinary temperature and pressure. Gases easily diffuse into other gases and they distribute throughout any container readily and uniformly.
4.  *Mist.* A finely divided liquid dispersed in air, which has been generated by mechanical agitation such as splashing, pouring or chemical reactions.
5.  *Vapor.* A gaseous state of a substance which is liquid or solid at ordinary temperature and pressure.

## RESPIRATORY HAZARD IDENTIFICATION
## AND EVALUATION

Proper identification of respiratory hazards and their evaluation is needed for several reasons, as noted on page 36.

Table 1.4  Site of action and pulmonary disease produced by selected occupationally inhaled toxicants

| TOXICANT | COMMON NAME OF DISEASE | SITE OF ACTION | ACUTE EFFECT | CHRONIC EFFECT |
|---|---|---|---|---|
| Asbestos | Asbestosis | Parenchyma | | Pulmonary fibrosis, pleural calcification, lung cancer, pleural mesothelioma |
| Aluminum | Aluminosis | Upper airways, alveolar interstitium | Cough, shortness of breath | Interstitial fibrosis |
| Aluminum abrasives | Shaver's disease, corundum smelter's lung, bauxite lung | Alveoli | Alveolar edema | Fibrotic thickening of alveolar walls, interstitial fibrosis and emphysema |
| Ammonia | | Upper airway | Immediate upper and lower respiratory tract irritation, edema | Chronic bronchitis |
| Arsenic | | Upper airways | Bronchitis | Lung cancer, bronchitis, laryngitis |
| Beryllium | Berylliosis | Alveoli | Severe pulmonary edema, pneumonia | Pulmonary fibrosis, progressive dyspnoea, interstitial granulomatosis, cor pulmonale |
| Boron | | Alveolus | Edema and hemorrhage | |
| Cadmium oxide | | Alveolus | Cough, pneumonia | Emphysema, cor pulmonale |
| Carbides of tungsten, titanium, tantalium | Hard metal disease | Upper airway and lower airway | Hyperplasia and metaplasia of bronchial epithelium | Fibrosis, peribronchial and perivascular fibrosis |

Table 1.4  *(continued)*

| TOXICANT | COMMON NAME OF DISEASE | SITE OF ACTION | ACUTE EFFECT | CHRONIC EFFECT |
|---|---|---|---|---|
| Chlorine | | Upper airways | Cough, hemoptysis, dyspnoea, tracheobronchitis, bronchopneumonia | |
| Chromium (VI) | | Nasopharynx, upper airways | Nasal irritation, bronchitis | Lung tumors and cancers |
| Coal dust | Pneumoconiosis | Lung paranchyma, lymph nodes, hilus | | Pulmonary fibrosis |
| Coke oven emissions | | Upper airways | | Tracheobronchial cancers |
| Cotton dust | Byssionsis | Upper airways | Tightness in chest, wheezing, dyspnea | Reduced pulmonary function, chronic bronchitis |
| Hydrogen fluoride | | Upper airways | Respiratory irritation, hemorrhagic pulmonary edema | |
| Iron oxides | Siderotic lung disease: Silver finisher's lung, hematite miner's lung, arc welder's lung | Silver finisher's pulmonary vessels and alveolar walls; hematite miner's: upper lobes, bronchi and alveoli; arc welder's; bronchi | Cough | Silver finisher's: subpleural and perivascular aggregations of macrophages; hematite miner's: diffuse fibrosis-like pneumoconiosis; arc welder's: bronchitis |
| Kaolin | Kaolinosis | Lung parenchyma, lymph nodes, hilus | | Pulmonary fibrosis |
| Manganese | Manganese pneumonia | Lower airways and alveoli | Acute pneumonia, often fatal | Recurrent pneumonia |
| Nickel | | Parenchyma (NiCO), nasal mucosa ($Ni_2S_3$), bronchi (NiO) | Pulmonary edema, delayed by 2 days (NiCO) | Squamous cell carcinoma of nasal cavity and lung |

| TOXICANT | COMMON NAME OF DISEASE | SITE OF ACTION | ACUTE EFFECT | CHRONIC EFFECT |
|---|---|---|---|---|
| Osmium tetraoxide | | Upper airways | Bronchitis, bronchopneumonia | |
| Oxides of nitrogen | | Terminal respiratory bronchi and alveoli | Pulmonary congestion and edema | Emphysema |
| Ozone | | Terminal respiratory bronchi and alveoli | Pulmonary edema | Emphysema |
| Phosgene | | Alveoli | Edema | Bronchitis |
| Perchloroethylene | | | Pulmonary edema | |
| Silica | Silicosis, pneumoconiosis | Lung parenchyma, lymph nodes, hilus | | Pulmonary fibrosis |
| Sulfur dioxide | | Upper airways | Bronchoconstriction, cough, tightness in chest | |
| Talc | Talcosis | Lung parenchyma, lymph nodes | | Pulmonary fibrosis |
| Tin | Stanosis | Bronchioles and pleura | | Widespread mottling of x-ray without clinical signs |
| Toluene | | Upper airways | Acute bronchitis, bronchospasm, pulmonary edema | |
| Vanadium | | Upper and lower airways | Upper airway irritation and mucus production | Chronic bronchitis |
| Xylene | | Lower airways | Pulmonary edema | |

(From J. Poull, C. Klaassen and M. Amdur, *Casarett and Doull's Toxicity* 1980, MacMillan Publishing Co. Inc., New York)

Table 1.5   Air contaminants from industrial processes

| PROCESS TYPE | CONTAMINANT TYPE | EXAMPLES OF CHEMICAL CONTAMINANTS |
|---|---|---|
| Abrasives (Manufacture) | Dust | aluminum oxide, silicon carbide silica, emery, corondum |
| | Gas/Vapours | carbon monoxide, solvent vapours from adhesives, vapourized resins |
| Adhesives (Manufacture and Use) | Vapours | solvent vapours, resins |
| Asphalt Paving | Dust | silica, silicates, carbonates |
| | Vapours | polycyclic aromatic hydrocarbons, aromatic and aliphatic hydrocarbon solvents |
| Automotive (Repair and Maintenance) | Dust/Fibres | asbestos, metal and resin dust from grinding |
| | Fumes | metal oxides (welding) |
| | Gas/Vapours | petroleum solvents, gasoline, carbon monoxide, hydrogen, nitrogen oxides, styrene, acetone, isocyanates, organic peroxides |
| Bakeries | Dust | flour, other vegetable dust, yeast, molds |
| Battery Manufacture | Dust/Fume | lead, cadmium |
| | Gas | hydrogen, formaldehyde, vinyl chloride |
| | Mists | sulfuric acid, hydrochloric acid, alkali mists |

Table 1.5   *(continued)*

| PROCESS TYPE | CONTAMINANT TYPE | EXAMPLES OF CHEMICAL CONTAMINANTS |
|---|---|---|
| Beverage and Soft Drink Manufacture | Gas | ammonia, carbon dioxide |
| | Mists | caustic mists |
| Blasting, Abrasive | Dust | silica, silicates, carbonates, lead, cadmium, zinc |
| Boiler Making | Dust | silicates, fluorides, carbonates |
| | Fume | welding fumes, metal fumes |
| Brewing | Gas | refrigerant gases, carbon dioxide |
| | Mist | caustic mists |
| Brick and Tile Manufacture | Dust | silica, silicates, fluorides, carbonates |
| | Gas (Kilns) | carbon monoxide |
| Business Machines (Photocopying and Duplicating) | Gas | ammonia, ozone |
| | Vapours | methyl alcohol, chlorinated hydrocarbons and petroleum solvents |
| Can Manufacture | Fumes | metal fumes |
| | Vapours | solvent vapours |
| Cement Manufacture | Dust | silica, silicates, fluorides, carbonates, chromates |

Table 1.5   *(continued)*

| PROCESS TYPE | CONTAMINANT TYPE | EXAMPLES OF CHEMICAL CONTAMINANTS |
|---|---|---|
| Cement Products Industry | Dust | cement |
|  | Fumes | welding fumes |
|  | Gas/Vapours | gasoline, acetone, lacquer thinner, kerosene, fuel oil, stoddard solvent |
| Charcoal Production | Gas | carbon monoxide, polycyclic aromatic hydrocarbons |
| Chemical Manufacture: Acid Plants | Gas | sulfur dioxide, nitrogen oxides |
|  | Mists | acid mists |
| Benzoic Acid | Dust | benzoic acid |
| Chlor-alkali Plant | Gas/Vapour | chlorine, mercury |
|  | Mist | sodium hydroxide |
| Fertilizer | Dust | fluoride, phosphate, silicates, carbonates, distomacious earth |
|  | Gas | ammonia, hydrogen fluoride |
|  | Mist | phosphoric acid |
| Solvents | Vapours | solvent vapours - alcohols, ketones, esters, aliphatic hydrocarbons, aromatic hydrocarbons, chlorinated hydrocarbons |

Table 1.5 *(continued)*

| PROCESS TYPE | CONTAMINANT TYPE | EXAMPLES OF CHEMICAL CONTAMINANTS |
|---|---|---|
| Clay | Dust | mica, silicates, iron oxide, silica (quartz) |
| Coal Handling | Dust | coal dust, silica |
| | Gas | sulfur dioxide, carbon monoxide |
| Coke Handling | Dust | coke dust |
| Coking | Gas | carbon monoxide, ammonia, hydrogen sulfide, sulfur dioxide, phenols, cyanides, naphthalene and other polycyclic aromatic hydrocarbons, benzene, pyridine, carbon disulfide |
| Dairy Processing Industry | Mist | alkali mists |
| Dental Industry | Vapour | mercury |
| Detergent Manufacture and use | Dusts | proteolytic enzymes, sodium perborate, phosphates |
| | Mists | alkali mists |
| Distilleries | Vapour | alcohol (ethyl alcohol) |
| Drilling (Rock) | Dust | silica, silicates, carbonates, fluorides |
| Dry Cleaning | Vapour | perchlorethylene, trichloroethylene, petroleum solvents |

Table 1.5   *(continued)*

| PROCESS TYPE | CONTAMINANT TYPE | EXAMPLES OF CHEMICAL CONTAMINANTS |
|---|---|---|
| Electrical Components Manufacturing Industry | Fumes | metal fumes (silver, lead, cadmium, tin) |
| | Vapours | solvent vapours, freon gases |
| Electroplating and Galvanizing Acid | Gas | hydrogen |
| | Mist | chromic acid, sulfuric acid, cyanide, sulfamate, hydrochloric acid, hydrofluoric acid |
| Alkaline | Gas | ammonia |
| | Mist | sodium stannate (tin salt) |
| Cyanide | Gas | ammonia, hydrogen cyanide |
| | Mist | cyanide, alkali |
| Electrodeless Plating | Gas | formaldehyde, ammonia |
| Electropolishing | Gas | hydrogen fluoride, hydrogen chloride |
| | Mist | sulfuric acid, hydrofluoric acid, phosphoric acid, hydrochloric acid, chromic acid, perchloric acid |
| Fluoroborate | Mist | fluoroborate mist |

Table 1.5  *(continued)*

| PROCESS TYPE | CONTAMINANT TYPE | EXAMPLES OF CHEMICAL CONTAMINANTS |
|---|---|---|
| Galvanizing | Dust | metal oxide |
| | Fumes | lead, zinc |
| | Gas | ammonia, hydrogen chloride |
| | Mist | alkali, hydrochloric acid, sulfuric acid |
| Explosives | Gas | oxides of nitrogen, carbon monoxide, sulfur dioxide |
| Fibreglassing (also see plastics) | Dust | asbestos, wood dust, glass fibres, resins, glycols, peroxides |
| | Vapours | acetone, styrene, amines, alcohols, phthalates, methyl ethyl ketone, toluene, phenol, isocyanates |
| Foundries, Furnaces and Forges<br>  Basic Oxygen Furnace<br>  Material Handling | Dust | iron oxide, graphite, limestone, ore, mill scale, fluorspar |
|   Forging | Gas | sulfur dioxide, carbon monoxide, carbon dioxide |
| | Vapour | acrolein |
| Foundry Operations | Dust | silica, silicates, carbonates, fluoride, cyanides |
| | Fumes | metal oxides |

Table 1.5    *(continued)*

| PROCESS TYPE | CONTAMINANT TYPE | EXAMPLES OF CHEMICAL CONTAMINANTS |
|---|---|---|
| | Gas | ammonia, carbon monoxide, sulfur dioxide phosgene, chlorine, fluorine, nitrogen oxides |
| | Vapours | acrolein, aldehydes, phenols, isocyanates, polycyclic aromatic hydrocarbons |
| Furnace Operations (all types) | Dust/Fumes | iron oxide, other metal oxides, fluxing agents |
| | Gas | sulfur dioxide, carbon monoxide, other combustion products |
| Leaded Steel Making | Dust/Fumes | lead oxide, iron oxide |
| Sintering | Dust | iron oxide, silica, fluorides, carbonates, metal oxides |
| | Gas | sulfur dioxide, carbon monoxide |
| Tandem Mills | Mist | oil mists |
| Frozen Food Industry | Gas | ammonia, methyl chloride, freons |
| Gases – Compressed | Gas | asphyxiating, corrosive or toxic gases, flammable or explosive gases |
| Glass Industry Etching | Gas | hydrogen fluoride |
| Fibreglassing (see fibreglassing) | | |

Table 1.5  *(continued)*

| PROCESS TYPE | CONTAMINANT TYPE | EXAMPLES OF CHEMICAL CONTAMINANTS |
|---|---|---|
| Manufacture | Dust/Fumes | silica, lead, soda ash, potash, vanadium, arsenic |
| | Fibres | asbestos |
| | Gas | sulfur dioxide, hydrogen fluoride |
| | Mist | oil mists |
| Hair and Bristle Processing Industry | Dust | fibre dust, spores of animal diseases |
| | Gas/Vapours | sulfur dioxide, hypochlorite vapour |
| Hospitals | Gas | formaldehyde, anesthetic gases, ethylene oxide |
| Insulation Manufacturing | Dust | mineral dust, cellulose dust, silica |
| | Fibres | asbestos, glass |
| | Vapours | isocyanates |
| Joineries, Cabinet Making and Furniture Manufacture | Dust | wood dust |
| | Vapours | solvents, glues, paints |
| Metal Cleaning & Surface Treatment Operations Abrasive Cleaners | Dust | silica, insoluble silicates, calcium carbonate, pumice, sodium carbonate, sodium silicate, di- and tri-sodium phosphate |

Table 1.5   *(continued)*

| PROCESS TYPE | CONTAMINANT TYPE | EXAMPLES OF CHEMICAL CONTAMINANTS |
|---|---|---|
| Acid cleaners dipping | Gas | oxides of nitrogen, hydrogen, hydrogen chloride |
| | Mist | nitric acid, sulfuric acid, chromic acid, hydrochloric acid |
| pickling | Gas | oxides of nitrogen, hydrogen fluoride, hydrogen chloride, hydrogen cyanide, hydrogen, arsine |
| Alkaline Cleaners | Mist | alkali mists |
| Case Hardening | Gas | carbon monoxide, oxygen deficiency, cyanides |
| Etching | Gas | hydrogen fluoride |
| | Mist | alkali mists |
| Degreasing | Vapours | trichlorethylene, perchloroethylene, petroleum and chlorinated hydrocarbon solvents |
| Strike Solutions | Gas | hydrogen chloride |
| | Mist | cyanide, chloride |
| Stripping Operations | Gas | hydrogen chloride, oxides of nitrogen |
| | Mist | hydrochloric acid, chromic acid, acetic acid, nitric acid, hydrofluoric acid, cyanide, alkali mists |

Table 1.5　*(continued)*

| PROCESS TYPE | CONTAMINANT TYPE | EXAMPLES OF CHEMICAL CONTAMINANTS |
|---|---|---|
| Metal Spraying | Dust/Fumes | metals and oxides of metals (eg. nickel, chromium, cobalt) |
| Paint Manufacture | Fumes | lead oxide, mercuric oxide resins |
| | Vapours | solvents, isocyanates, polyurethanes, insecticide |
| Paperboard/Container Industry | Fumes | welding fumes |
| | Gas | formaldehyde, carbon monoxide |
| | Vapours | gasoline, acetone, lacquer thinner, kerosene, fuel oil, stoddard solvent |
| Pest Control Fungicides, Herbicides Pesticides, Rodenti- cides | Dust/Vapours | organophosphorus compounds, halo- genated hydrocarbons, lead arsenate, carbonates, thiocarbonates, dinitrocresol, thallium and its compounds, coumarin, indane and derivatives, chloropicrin, mercury, creosote, dinitrophenol, solvents |
| Petroleum Refineries | Gas | hydrogen sulfide, mercaptans, liquified petroleum gases |
| | Vapours | solvent vapours |
| Photographic Industry | Dust | organic dyes |
| | Vapours | aminophenols, hydroquinone, acetic acid |

Table 1.5   *(continued)*

| PROCESS TYPE | CONTAMINANT TYPE | EXAMPLES OF CHEMICAL CONTAMINANTS |
|---|---|---|
| Plastics and Resins | Gas | thermal decomposition products, (carbon monoxide, carbon dioxide, oxides of nitrogen), blowing agents |
| | Vapours | isocyanates, monomers (eg. styrene, vinyl chloride) |
| Plumbing, Heating and Air Conditioning Contractors | Fibres | asbestos, glass |
| | Fumes | welding fumes |
| | Gas | carbon monoxide, refrigeration gases |
| | Mist | acid mists, caustic mists |
| | Vapours | solvents |
| Pottery and Porcelain Industry | Dust | clay, silica, silicates |
| | Fumes | lead |
| Power Stations (thermal) | Dust | vanadium oxide, nickel |
| | Gas | sulfur dioxide |
| | Mist | oil |
| Printing | Dust/Fumes | lead, chromium compounds, antimony, nickel salts |

Table 1.5   *(continued)*

| PROCESS TYPE | CONTAMINANT TYPE | EXAMPLES OF CHEMICAL CONTAMINANTS |
|---|---|---|
| | Mist | chromic acid, alkalis |
| | Vapours | solvents (turpentine, benzene, toluene, xylene, alcohols) |
| Pulp and Paper Industry Bleaching | Gas | chlorine, chlorine dioxide, sulfur dioxide |
| Chlorine Dioxide Generation | Gas | sulfur dioxide, chlorine dioxide, chlorine |
| | Mist | sulfuric acid mist |
| Digesting | Gas | methyl mercaptan, dimethyl sulfide, dimethyl disulfide, hydrogen sulfide |
| Lime Kiln | Dust | calcium oxide, calcium carbonate, sodium oxide |
| | Gas | carbon dioxide |
| | Mist | alkali mist |
| Recovery Furnaces | Dust | sodium sulfate |
| | Gas | carbon dioxide, sulfur dioxide, hydrogen sulfide, mercaptans |
| Refrigeration Plants | Gas | ammonia, hydrogen chloride, ethane, chlorine, methyl chloride, phosgene, sulfur dioxide, ethyl chloride, propane, butane, ethylene, freons |

Table 1.5   *(continued)*

| PROCESS TYPE | CONTAMINANT TYPE | EXAMPLES OF CHEMICAL CONTAMINANTS |
|---|---|---|
| Rock Crushing and Drilling | Dust | silica, silicates, carbonates, fluorides |
| | Gas | internal combustion engine exhaust gases - oxides of nitrogen, sulfur dioxide, carbon monoxide, aldehydes |
| Roofing Industry | Dust/Fibres | asbestos, cement dust |
| | Fumes | metal oxides |
| | Vapours | solvents, asphalt |
| Rubber Industry Synthetic | Mist | acetic acid, sulfuric acid |
| | Vapours | acrylonitrile, benzene, butadiene, chloro-butadiene, isocyanates, styrene, ethyl benzene, isoprene, dichloroethane |
| Vulcanizing | Gas | sulfur dioxide |
| | Vapour | organic solvents |
| Sawmilling and Planing Filing Room | Dust/Fumes | cadmium, metals, metal oxide, mineral dust, welding fumes |
| | Fibres | asbestos |
| Wood Rooms | Dust | wood dust |
| | Mist | oil mist |

Table 1.5   *(continued)*

| PROCESS TYPE | CONTAMINANT TYPE | EXAMPLES OF CHEMICAL CONTAMINANTS |
|---|---|---|
| Scrap Metal Processors | Fumes | lead, cadmium, mercury, zinc, welding fumes |
| | Gas | fluorine |
| | Vapours | solvents |
| Sewage Disposal and Treatment | Gas | methane, carbon dioxide, hydrogen sulfide, mercaptans |
| Sewers | Gas | oxygen deficiency, methane, carbon monoxide, hydrogen sulfide, carbon dioxide, liquified petroleum gases |
| | Vapours | gasoline, petroleum solvents |
| Shipbuilding | Dust/Fibres | asbestos, metal oxides |
| | Fumes | lead, organotin and organomercurial anti-fouling paints, welding fumes |
| | Gas | combustion products (carbon monoxide, oxides of nitrogen) |
| Sign and Advertising Display Manufacturers | Fibres | asbestos |
| | Fumes | welding fumes |
| | Vapours | methylene chloride, methyl ethyl ketone, methanol, xylene, mercury |

Table 1.5   *(continued)*

| PROCESS TYPE | CONTAMINANT TYPE | EXAMPLES OF CHEMICAL CONTAMINANTS |
|---|---|---|
| Silos | Gas | oxygen deficiency, oxides of nitrogen |
| Slaughtering Plants (Digesters and Rendering) | Dust | sodium hydroxide, sodium carbonate |
| | Gas | chlorine, refrigerant gases |
| | Mist | sulfuric acid, phosphoric acid, acetic acid |
| | Vapours | formaldehyde, phenol or cresol based sanitizers |
| Smelting and Refining | Dust/Fumes | metal oxides, selenium, tellurium, cadmium, arsenic, lead, bismuty, indium, silver, gold, fluoride, metal fumes and dusts |
| | Gas | arsine, sulfur dioxide, carbon monoxide, hydrogen selenide, hyrdogen fluoride |
| | Mist | sulfuric acid, fluorosilicic acid |
| Soldering | Fumes | metal fumes (silver, cadmium, lead, tin) |
| | Vapours | formaldehyde, acrolein, aldehydes |
| Sterilization Processes | Gas | ozone, ethylene oxide, halogenated hydrocarbons |

Table 1.5   *(continued)*

| PROCESS TYPE | CONTAMINANT TYPE | EXAMPLES OF CHEMICAL CONTAMINANTS |
|---|---|---|
| Tunnelling (underground) | Dust | silica, silicates, fluorides, carbonates |
| | Gas | internal combustion engine exhaust gases, oxygen deficiency, oxides of nitrogen, carbon monoxide, natural gases (methane), sulfur dioxide, aldehydes, explosive by-products |
| Water Supply and Treatment | Gas | chlorine, ammonia, hydrogen chloride, ozone |
| | Mist | hydrochloric acid, sodium hydroxide, calcium hydroxide |
| Welding and Thermal Cutting | Dust/Fumes | metal oxides, welding fumes, silicates, carbonates, fluorspar, metal fumes, fluoride |
| | Gas | oxides of nitrogen, ozone, phosgene, carbon monoxide, hydrogen fluoride |
| Wineries | Gas | carbon dioxide, refrigerant gases, sulfur dioxide |
| | Vapour | ethyl alcohol |
| Wood Processing and Treatment   Wood Treatment | Dust | arsenic and copper compounds |
| | Vapours | pentachlorophenol, tetrachlorophenol |

Table 1.5    *(continued)*

| PROCESS TYPE | CONTAMINANT TYPE | EXAMPLES OF CHEMICAL CONTAMINANTS |
|---|---|---|
| Plywood and Veneer Mills<br>    Filing Room | Dust/Fibres | metal dust (cadmium, tin, antimony, copper, lead), asbesotos |
| Maintenance Shops | Fumes | welding fumes |
| | Gas | carbon monoxide, nitrogen oxides |
| Paint and Stains | Vapours | organic solvents, pigments (compounds of titanium, iron, lead, cadmium, chromium) |
| Sawing and Sanding | Dust | wood dust, wood preservatives |
| Veneer Drying<br>Glueing & Patching | Dust | resins, catalysts |
| | Gas | ammonia, formaldehyde |
| | Vapours | isocyanates, methylene chloride, urea, phenol, terpenes, alcohols, aldehydes, esters, ketones |

1.  To determine the extent of exposure to the toxic substances,
2.  To demonstrate compliance with the legal exposure limits,
3.  To assess the effectiveness of engineering and administrative controls, and
4.  To determine if the level or concentration indicates the need for additional respiratory protection.

In addition, this information is also used for the correct selection of respirators for specific toxic substances listed earlier.

Hazards are usually identified by conducting a preliminary survey. The purpose of this survey is to document the materials used or produced, how they are handled, general working conditions, and the persons who may be exposed to a hazard.

The variety of materials in the workplace includes all the raw materials, products and by-products, depending upon the process, the exposures to any or all of these substances could be important. For example, paint thinner is a raw material in paint manufacturing. A spray-painter is therefore exposed to paint thinner vapors. Undesirable reaction products are formed during certain process operations, such as the formation of zinc oxide fumes during the welding and torch-cutting of galvanized steel. Another example is the inadvertent breakdown of chemical compounds into more toxic substances, such as the formation of phosgene gas by welding near a vapor degreaser containing trichloroethylene solvent.

Recognizing a hazard is made easier if pure chemicals are used in the process. When proprietary mixtures of chemicals are encountered, the identification of a hazard may be difficult if the manufacturer is not willing to supply information on the products. Having compiled an inventory of raw materials, products and by-products, it would then be necessary to review the relevant toxicological information outlined in the Material Safety Data Sheets (M.S.D.S.).

## THE EVALUATION PROCESS

After the completion of a preliminary survey, which is accomplished in a day or less, an environmental evaluation of worker exposure to airborne contaminants may be required. The evaluation can be made in two different ways:

1. By sampling the worker's respiratory zone, usually accomplished by "personal sampling," i.e., the worker is required to wear a personal sampling head and pump to determine the concentration of contaminants to which he/she is exposed (Figure 1.7).
2. By sampling the workplace air referred to as "area sampling."

In recent years, personal sampling has become more popular because it gives the best estimate of worker exposure, taking into account parameters such as time and space fluctuations, and different tasks performed during the shift.

The area sample, on the other hand, is collected to measure the amount of air contaminant to which the worker is exposed. The source of contamination may or may not be associated with what the people are doing in the area. However, if the airborne concentration in an area is expected to remain fairly constant, then area samples may be used for estimating personal exposures.

## SAMPLING EQUIPMENT

Figure 1.8 shows the components of a personal sampling unit which consists of:

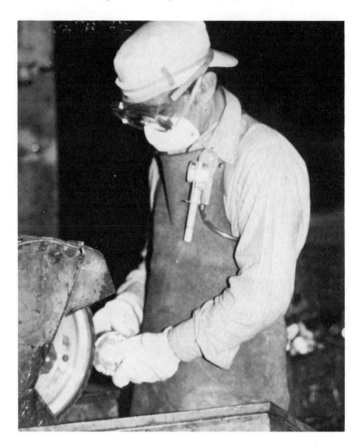

**Figure 1.7**  Personal air sampling.

1.  A sampling head on a collection device such as a filter, tube, or impinger which includes a component that can trip or react to the contaminant being measured;
2.  A flowmeter which indicates the rate of airflow through the sampler; and
3.  A pump or other suction device to draw environmental air.

The following accessories are available with the above-mentioned basic equipment:

1.  *Pulsation damper.* Pulsation in the pump may interfere with proper functioning of the sampling intake, especially if the latter has, for instance, a particle-size selector cyclone. A narrower chamber with flexible walls situated in series in the pump circuit acts as a capacity to

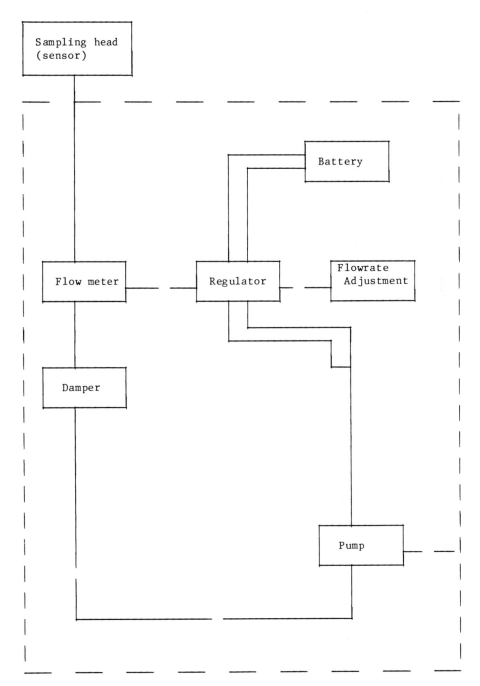

**Figure 1.8** Components of a personal sampling unit.

damp pulsations in flowrate. This device has been incorporated in nearly all personal dust-sampling devices.

2. *Flowrate regulation devices.* The sampling of workplace air necessitates a relatively constant flowrate, especially for some types of particle-size reactors, the dimensions of which are calculated for a certain flowrate, and their efficiency is closely linked to a constant flowrate. Constant flowrate is also necessary to avoid gross errors in determining the volume sampled.

To overcome these problems, sampling instruments usually have a compensating device to limit the effects of variations in pressure upstream from the pump caused by progressive clogging of the filter.

There are several types of direct-reading instruments available to determine contaminant concentrations in air. Comprehensive information on these instruments is available in *Air Sampling Instruments* for evaluation of atmospheric contaminants, published by the American Conference of Governmental Industrial Hygienists (ACGIH) [3]. These instruments read out the concentration of a collected sample directly without needing any elaborate laboratory analysis, and feature detector tubes, direct-reading gas monitors, direct-reading dust monitors and mercury vapor meters. The most popular among them are detector tubes.

A detector tube consists of a hand pump, a detector tube and a calibrated scale or color standard. The detector tube is a sealed glass tube containing a solid support inpregnated with a reactive chemical reagent. An air sample is drawn through the tube with a hand pump, and if a contaminant is present, it reacts with the reagent in the tube producing a color. This color represents the level of concentration of the contaminant in the air.

NIOSH-certified detector tubes are accurate to ± 35% at 1/2 the TLV and ± 25% at 1.0, 2, and 5 times the TLV if tubes are stored according to the manufacturer's instructions. Thus, the tubes are good indicators of very high and very low concentrations. In the range of 20%, variation above or below the health standard the tubes lack the accuracy required in making a decision. In this "gray area," samples should be taken using the sampling train described above.

Another problem with detector tubes is the lack of specificity. Many tubes are far from specific, and hence, accurate knowledge of the possible interfering gases cannot be obtained. In order to quantify the effect of these present interfering gases, and to avoid dangerously misleading results, the interpretation of detector tube measurements must be supervised by a qualified industrial hygienist.

There are several battery-operated gas monitors available, including monitors for carbon monoxide, hydrogen sulfide, combustible gases, organic vapors and oxygen. The theory, principles of operation and application of these instruments are well documented in the ACGIH literature [3]. Some of these instruments are based on the principle of electrical conductivity; that chemical or physical properties of gas contaminants introduce variations in the electrical parameters of the input sensor so that the sensor output is related to the concentration of the gas being measured.

Other direct reading gas monitors use the principle of infrared photometry (e.g., IRCO analyzer), mass spectroscopy (e.g., $SO_2$ analyzer), and ultraviolet photometry (e.g., mercury vapor analyzer).

All this equipment is limited in its application and use because it is essentially non-specific for one contaminant, and secondly, it takes grab samples. Thus, it suffers from the same disadvantages as the detector tubes. It has been suggested that a series of grab samples may be used to determine the time-weighted averages over a long period of time, however, this involves careful planning regarding sampling strategy and the treatment of the sampling results obtained.

There are very few reliable direct-reading monitors available. They include the digital-dust indicator, the "Royco" particle counter, the respirable-dust mass monitor and the fibrous-aerosol monitor. The principle involved in their use is the passing of an aerosol through a sensing region. The pressure of the particle gives rise to the detection of a change in a property of the region. A simple relationship is established between the detected change and a property of the aerosol.

Different aerosol properties are measured by different direct-reading instruments, hence the properties may not be directly compared without some modifications of the data to account for the differences. Some of the properties determined include particle sizes, aerosol number concentrations and aerosol mass concentrations.

The accuracy of these instruments is generally limited because it depends upon the relationship between the sensing region, and aerosol property is based on an empirical formula using a "well-calibrated" aerosol system. The real aerosol measure may have a different, unknown relationship.

Another type of air-monitoring device is the diffusional monitor. It operates on the principle of diffusion, which is a process by which vapors and gases flow from high concentrations in the workplace to near zero concentrations inside the monitor. The driving force for the sampling is the concentration gradient between the face of the monitor and the sorbent layer in the monitor. Air sampling with diffusional monitors provides a convenient and economical test of air quality in a worker's breathing zone. Diffusional monitors are easy to wear, simple to use and highly accurate. More details can be found in Rose and Perkins' review article published in 1982 [4].

## SAMPLING PROCEDURE AND SAMPLING STRATEGY

Air sampling involves drawing air through a collection device at a known flow rate. The quantity of substance gathered on the device is then determined through laboratory analysis. From this information, and the known quantity of air which has been drawn through the sampler, it is possible to calculate the concentration of substance in the sampled air. In order to collect representative samples, it is essential to consider the following:

1. The duration of sampling,
2. When to conduct the sampling,
3. The number of samples, and
4. The frequency of sampling.

The duration of sampling (i.e., the amount of time involved in drawing air through the sampling device) will depend on the type of exposure concentration being measured. The recommended minimum sampling duration varies from contaminant to contaminant. When determining the time-weighted average exposure concentration, sampling is usually conducted for 6 to 8 hours, or for a full work shift. However, a shorter sampling time may be used if it is planned to reflect representative exposure levels.

When determining compliance with the maximum allowable exposure level, a series of 15 minute samples should be taken during time periods when maximum emissions are expected.

In most industrial operations there are fluctuations in the concentration of contaminants in the air. Before establishing a sampling strategy, it is important to have thoroughly evaluated the nature of the operation in order to determine when, and under what conditions, the substance may be emitted. Representative sampling times should then be chosen so that it will be possible to calculate exposure over a full work week. For example, if operations do not vary from day to day, it will probably be sufficient to base calculations of weekly exposure on full-shift sampling conducted for one day. If there is considerable daily variation, then sampling should be conducted over several days, representing the different exposure conditions. If exposure conditions vary from week to week, sampling should be performed during a week when maximum exposure is expected.

The number of samples gathered should be planned to obtain a representative picture of exposure conditions. In order to compensate for errors inherent in sampling and analysis procedures, it is generally expected that a minimum of three samples will be gathered for each exposure situation. This may be done by taking separate samples, under similar exposure conditions, at the same time; it may also be done by sampling, in the same location, under the same exposure conditions, on different days.

The number of samples to be collected may also depend upon the operations being studied and whether the TLV is a time-weighted average, a ceiling value, or both.

The frequency with which air sampling is done is based on the exposure conditions in the individual work place. If exposure levels are regularly near the allowable limits, air monitoring will be necessary more often. In such cases, monitoring may be appropriate on a monthly or quarterly basis. Where exposure levels are usually much lower than prescribed limits, semi-annual monitoring should be sufficient. However, air sampling should always be performed when there are any changes in the process or conditions of exposure.

Sampling must be conducted by personnel, e.g., an industrial hygienist who is trained to operate monitoring devices and accurately record essential information. If frequent monitoring is necessary, the employer may want to hire staff trained in sampling techniques, or train employees who are already on staff. If this is not desirable, the employer may contract with private consultants to conduct air-monitoring tests, or he may ask for assistance from a safety association.

In most situations, employers will send the samples they have collected to a public or private chemical laboratory for analysis. In choosing a lab, the employer must ascertain that it will analyze the samples according to the standard methods and procedures.

Time-Weighted Average Exposure Levels (TWAEL) refer to the maximum average exposure of a worker during an 8-hour day or 40-hour week. These levels are commonly referred to as Threshold-Limit Values or TLVs published and updated annually by the American Conference of Governmental Industrial Hygienists (ACGIH) [5]. Several countries have adopted these values giving them legal status in their health and safety regulations, despite a warning from the ACGIH. In order to determine the time-weighted average exposure for comparison with the TWAEL, it is essential that samples taken represent exposure conditions over the course of a day. The results of analysis give the airborne concentration of the substance during this time. From this information the 8 hour time-weighted average exposure concentration can be determined by multiplying the concentrates $C_1$ by the time $T_1$ hours in which the worker is exposed to such concentration, and dividing the cumulative daily exposure by 8. This may be expressed as:

$$\frac{C_1T_1 + C_2T_2 + \ldots + C_nT_n}{8}$$

The basic difference between short-term exposures and ceiling values is that short-term levels are specified time-weighted average maximum or values for 15 minutes whereas ceiling values are the maximum values at any time.

The air samples obtained for both short-term and ceiling values are usually taken for a much shorter period of time than those taken for calculating the time-weighted averages. Each measurement usually consists of a 15 minute sample (or series of sequential samples totaling 15 minutes) or an instantaneous air sample.

There may be occasions when the interday variations in exposure appear minimal because of the very nature of the work process or operation.

In such cases, additional measurements should be made to ensure that there will be one or more sampling periods during which the maximum concentrations can be detected.

Since no sample measurement gives an absolute, correct answer and every sample differs from the respective true average concentration, statistical methods are used to calculate interval limits for each side of the average-exposure concentration at a selected statistical confidence level (e.g., 95%). The numerically larger limit is known as the Upper Confidence Limit (UCL) and the numerically lower limit is known as the Lower Confidence Limit (LCL). The UCL and LCL are calculated differently depending upon the type of air-sampling strategy used and the number of air samples taken to derive the average-exposure estimate. These levels are also related to the total coefficient of variation, $Cv_T$, for the sampling and analytical methods. For tests which comply with the legal standard promulgated in a country or state, the following steps are generally followed:

1.  If the lower confidence limit of the exposure estimate exceeds the exposure limit or criterion, we can be 95% confident that the exposure limit or criterion has been exceeded (i.e., non-compliance).
2.  If the upper confidence limit of the exposure estimate does not exceed the exposure limit or criterion, we can be 95% confident that the exposure limit or criterion has not been exceeded (i.e., compliance).
3.  We cannot be 95% confident that the exposure limit or criterion is in compliance or non-compliance (i.e., no decision) for the following cases:
    a.  The exposure estimate does not exceed the exposure limit or criterion but the upper confidence limit of the exposure estimate exceeds the exposure limit or criterion.
    b.  The exposure estimate exceeds the exposure limit or criterion but the lower confidence limit of the exposure estimate does not exceed the exposure limit or criterion.

In case no decision can be reached, further air sampling or appropriate statistical analyses should be considered and the workplace should be made aware of the possibility of exposure to toxicants. For appropriate statistical analyses, readers may consult several good references listed at the end of the chapter [6,7,8].

The respiratory tract is a very sensitive system in the human body and it is assaulted daily by numerous contaminants which can cause harm to the respiratory tract itself or other vital organs of the body. It is essential that one be aware of the nature and levels of contaminants in the air. This chapter has summarized the different airborne hazardous materials and methods available to determine their concentration in the workplace.

## REFERENCES

1. Olishifski, J.B., *Fundamentals of Industrial Hygiene,* 2nd Ed., National Safety Council, Chapter 2 (1979).
2. Poull, J., Klaassen, C., and Amdur, M., *Casarett and Doull's Toxicity,* MacMillan Publishing Co., Inc., New York (1980).
3. "Air Sampling Instruments for Evaluation of Atmospheric Contaminants," American Conference of Governmental Industrial Hygienists, 6th Ed., Cincinnati (1984).
4. Rose, V.E. and Perkins, J.L., "Passive Dosimetry—State of the Art Review." American Industrial Hygiene Association Journal, 43(8) (1982):605–621.
5. "TLVs® Threshold Limit Values for Chemical Substances and Physical Agents in the Work Environment with Intended Changes for 1983–84," American Conference of Governmental Industrial Hygienists, Cincinnati (1983).
6. Leidel, N.A., Busch, K.A., and Lynch, J.R., National Institute of Occupational Safety and Health, "Occupational Exposure Sampling Strategy Manual," U.S. Department of Health, Education and Welfare (NIOSH) Publication 77–173, (1977).
7. *Occupational Exposure Sampling Strategy Manual,* DHEW (NIOSH) Publication No. 77–173, (1977).
8. *Handbook of Statistical Tests for Evaluating Employee Exposure to Air Contaminants,* DHEW (NIOSH) Publication No. 75–147, (1975).

# 2

# *Respirator Types and Limitations*

Workers can be exposed to a large number of potential health hazards which may present an immediate or long term threat to them. Inhalation of airborne contaminants provides toxic materials the most direct access to the body and also provides a means to distribute them to other areas of the body. There are two types of respiratory hazards, namely airborne contaminants and oxygen deficiency.

Normal air contains 20.9% oxygen by volume. Concentrations below 16% are considered unsafe and can lead to death. Oxygen deficiency can be caused by gas and vapor displacement in a confined space. Workplace air should be maintained at a minimum of 19.5% oxygen. If the oxygen content is reduced to below 19.5%, for whatever reason, proper respiratory protection will be required.

Airborne contaminants can take different forms, such as dust, mist, gas, vapor, etc. Their effects on the human body can range from irritants to systemic poisons.

Under most occupational health and safety regulations, the health of workers must be protected by the use of engineering controls, and respirators should be used as a last resort. Typically, respirators are permitted under five conditions:

1.  To reduce exposure during the time needed to install engineering controls,
2.  To supplement engineering controls and work practices which fail to completely reduce the hazard to a permissible exposure level,
3.  During activities such as maintenance and repairs, when engineering controls are not feasible,
4.  During emergencies, and
5.  When measures and procedures necessary to control the exposure do not exist or are unavailable.

Engineering controls are by far the best method for effective and reliable protection from hazardous materials because they act to control the source of emission. Respirators, on the other hand, do not eliminate the hazard. But because of the five situations described above, a larger worker population must rely on respirators for necessary protection.

In order to ensure proper protection for workers, the correct respirator must be selected and the employer and worker must understand the limitations of each type of respirator. This chapter summarizes the different types of respirators available and the limitations of each.

Respirators can be classified into two main types: Air-Purifying and Atmosphere-Supplying.

## AIR-PURIFYING RESPIRATORS

Air-purifying respirators (Figure 2.1) are designed to remove contaminants in the form of particulates, gases and vapors, or combinations of all of these. The composition of the filtering medium depends on the contaminant to be filtered: various chemicals are used to remove specific gases and vapors while mechanical filters remove particulate matter. Within this classification, there are four basic types of air-purifying devices:

1.    Mechanical-Filter (Particulate) Respirator
2.    Chemical-Cartridge Respirator

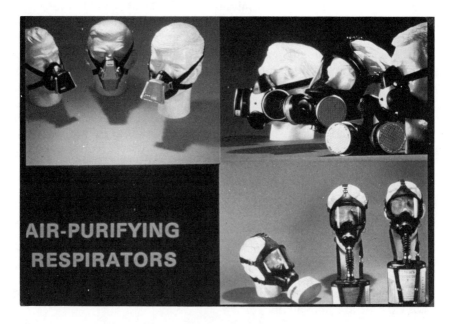

**Figure 2.1**  Air-purifying respirators: *Top left*—mechanical-filter type; *top right*—chemical cartridge type; *bottom right*—gas mask type.

3.  Gas Mask
4.  Powered Air-Purifying Respirator

## Mechanical-Filter Respirators

The mechanical-filter respirator provides respiratory protection against particulate matter such as dust, mist and fumes. Usually a fibrous material is used to trap the particulates, and its efficiency is dependent upon the size of the particle relative to the filter size, particle velocity and, to some extent, the composition and shape of both the particle and fiber. Figure 2.2 shows several different types of mechanical-filter respirators, from disposable to dual-cartridge type.

The mechanism of filtration can be either simple straining or depth filtration. Straining depends upon the solid particles being collected because they are larger than the pores in the medium. Depth filtration depends upon the particles adhering to the exposed surface of the filter medium within its depth. This type of filtration operates on a combination of mechanical and electrical forces, namely: interception, impaction, diffusion, and electrostatic. The specific type of force will depend mainly upon the particle size.

As air flows through a filter, the presence of fibers results in a curvature of the streamlines in the vicinity of the fiber. Very small particles, less then 0.01 microns in size, will not be carried by the air current. Brownian Motion, or diffusion, controls their movement, and eventually this random

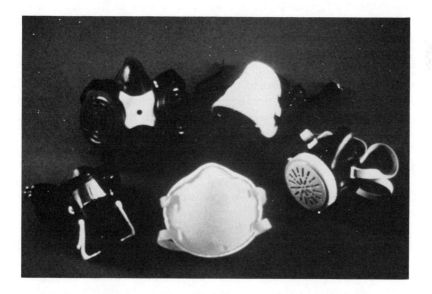

**Figure 2.2**  Different types of mechanical-filter respirators.

movement results in a collision with a solid surface. With decreasing particle size, diffusion becomes more intense and as a result the intensity of diffusional deposition increases. This mechanism is most significant in the removal of fine dusts. Larger particles may be trapped either through impaction or interception. Impaction will occur when a particle, because of its momentum, crosses the streamlines and impinges on the fiber. The frequency of impaction will increase with increasing particle size, and the velocity of flow, and it may also be referred to as inertial interception. Direct interception occurs when a particle is intercepted as it approaches the collecting surface at a distance equal to its radius. Figure 2.3 illustrates each of these filtering forces and a paper by D.A. Japuntich gives an excellent detailed explanation of these filtration mechanisms [1].

Electrostatic action is extremely important for removing small particles. Fibers and particles have electrical charges and generally increasing the charges on either of the two increases the opportunity for collecting the particle. The electrical charge generates a force which helps the particle move from the air streamline to a nearby fiber. A particle can move more than one radius across the air stream to a charged fiber (Figure 2.4). The fibers of a filter can be charged to influence particle collection. The wool resin filter, in which an electrostatic charge is developed when the wool and resin are carded together on a clothing machine, has been available since World War II. The main disadvantage of this filter medium is that the charge on the fibers is not always stable and will decrease with time.

Another development is the electret-fibrous filter. An electret is plastic with electrostatic charges physically embedded into the surface, which is then formed into a fibrous blanket. They can be seen as the electrical counterparts of magnets, i.e., they consist of dielectrics carrying a strong positive and negative electric charge.

For many years electrets have been considered a curiosity, but with large scale polymer production, they have found many applications. They are used in microphones because their natural charge requires no external power source; in fibrous-filter media which have been developed by Van Turnhout in the Netherlands and also by the firm of Carl Freudenberg in West Germany [2].

The bipolar charged electret fibers not only attract charged, but also uncharged particles. Charged particles are attracted by a strong coulombic force. Uncharged particles are polarized by the strong field around the electret fibers and converted to macroscopic dipoles and therefore attracted to the fibers.

The advantage of electrical forces over mechanical ones in trapping particulates is that electrical forces are active at some distance from the fibers. As a result, filters made from electrets have a rather open structure with large spaces, even if minute, sub-micron particles are captured efficiently. The open structure allows a stream of dust-laden air to pass through very easily so that the air resistance of electret filters is low, even at fairly high flow rates.

**Figure 2.3**   Filtration mechanisms.

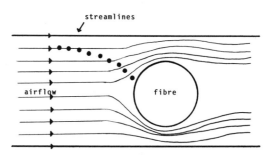

## SEDIMENTATION

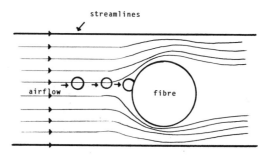

## IMPACTION

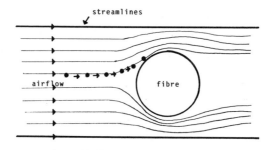

## INTERCEPTION

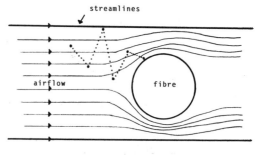

## DIFFUSION

**Figure 2.4** Electrostatic filtration mechanism.

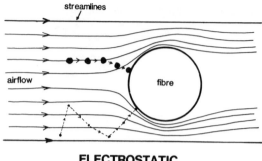

**ELECTROSTATIC**

The mechanical-filter or particulate-removing respirator group is generally called dust, mist or fume respirators, or combinations thereof. All dust, fume and mist respirators protect in exactly the same way, by removing and retaining the airborne particulate, before it can be inhaled. The mechanical-filter itself is generally composed of wool or a synthetic fiber. It may also consist of a filter composed of a resin-impregnated blend to which an electrostatic charge is imparted in order to increase its efficiency by electrostatically attracting the particles to the fibers.

No filter is 100% efficient in removing particles, and the probability that a single particle will be trapped depends on a multitude of factors, including the composition and shape of both the particle and the fiber. Hence, mechanical filters are also classified as designed for protection against dust, mists, fumes, and any combination thereof. For example, "toxic dust" filters are designed for protection against toxic dusts whose threshold limit value (TLV) is 0.05 MG/M³ or more. Some of these filters are also approved for mists whose TLV is 0.05 MG/M³ or more. "Fume" filters on the other hand are approved for contaminants, such as metal fumes, whose TLV is 0.05 MG/M³ or more, but have a higher efficiency toward particles less than 1 μm in diameter. Fume filters are generally accepted as being 99.5% efficient against 0.6 μm particles as opposed to 99.0% for dust filters. High-efficiency filters are designed to protect against particulate contaminants with a TLV less than 0.05 MG/M³ and are at least 99.97% efficient against 0.3 μm particles. High-efficiency filters, however, have poorer particle-loading characteristics, which tend to increase breathing resistance.

There are two basic designs of mechanical-filter respirators: cartridge and disposable (Figure 2.5). The cartridge respirator consists of a molded rubber or plastic facepiece which, when placed on the face, makes a seal between the skin and the molded facepiece. The cartridges, which act as the filtering medium, are screwed onto the facepiece. Cartridges are available for protection against particulates, gases/vapors, or combinations of the two. The cartridges are replaced when they are used up. In contrast to the cartridge-type respirator, disposable respirators have non-replaceable parts.

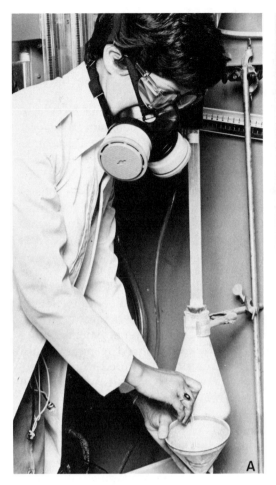
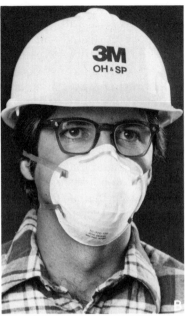

**Figure 2.5**  *A.* Cartridge-mechanical-filter respirator—Wilson Series 30 Stacked Cartridges (courtesy of Safety Supply Canada); *B.* Disposable mechanical-filter respirator—3M Brand Toxic Dust/Mist Respirator #8710 (courtesy of 3M Canada).

The entire respirator is disposed of when it is no longer usable. This eliminates the need for a maintenance program.

Depending on NIOSH approval, disposable respirators may be considered as *single use* or *replaceable* [3]. A single-use respirator refers to a specific certification granted by NIOSH. A disposable respirator can have NIOSH certification for single use, dust, mist, fume, high efficiency or chemical cartridge. Single-use and disposable are not equivalent descriptive terms for respiratory equipment. Single use refers to respirators approved by NIOSH for use against lung damaging dusts only, and must meet the requirements as specified in Federal Register 30-CFR-11. Replaceable refers to respirators which can be reused. That is, they can be removed and put back on and still will provide the necessary protection. These replaceable respirators are tested and must pass the requirements outlined in 30-CFR-11. Both the cartridge-type and the replaceable-disposable-type provide the same protection because both are considered replaceable and pass the same NIOSH test criteria (Summarized in Table 2.1).

There are two criteria used for replacing a dust/mist/fume respirator, or combinations thereof. First, the respirator or filter medium is damaged. Second, the filter or respirator is difficult to breathe through. Damage to the respirator or filter is usually very evident and thus the wearer is able to easily determine that the respirator or filter must be replaced.

The second criterion is much more difficult to determine. As the inhaled air is filtered, the particles build-up in the filter medium and clog the pores. This results in increasing breathing resistance. Eventually resistance reaches a point where the wearer finds breathing very uncomfortable and the filter must be discarded.

The concentration of dust being filtered, the breathing rate of the wearer, the tolerance of the wearer, the loading characteristic of the filter, and the breathing resistance of the filter before loading, influence the length of time required to reach an uncomfortable breathing resistance.

Table 2.1 summarizes the NIOSH pressure drop requirements before and after testing which the NIOSH particulate-approved respirator must meet. Since all approved particulate respirators are required to pass these tests, loading characteristics may be similar to each other because they will be no worse than the NIOSH resistance requirements.

There is no accurate method of predetermining the service-life of a particulate respirator. The concentration of airborne dust is the major factor influencing service life. The more dust in the air the more dust the filter must be able to retain, and the faster it will clog. The breathing rate of the wearer will also influence the service-life. If a worker is doing light work, his breathing rate is approximately 20 liters/minute. If the workload is heavy the breathing rate may be 60 liters/minute or higher. This results in approximately three times the volume of air going through the filter and thus three times as much dust to be filtered and retained in the filter.

Mechanical-filter respirators are usually available in three different categories: quarter-face, half-face, and full-face (Figure 2.6). The quarter-face covers the mouth and nose; the half-face covers the mouth, nose and chin; the full-face respirator covers the face from the chin to the hairline and from ear to ear.

Proper selection of the correct mechanical-filter respirator will afford the worker protection from nuisance dust, toxic dusts, mists, fumes or any combinations, but there are important limitations:

1. They do not provide oxygen, so they must not be used in oxygen-deficient atmospheres.

Table 2.1   Dust, fume, mist respirators—summary of NIOSH tests

I – QUALITATIVE FACE FIT

(i) For air contamination levels not less than 0.05 mg/m$^3$
2 min. in 100 ppm of isoamyl acetate.

(ii) For air contamination levels less than 0.05 mg/m$^3$

half mask – 5 min. in 100 ppm of isoamyl acetate
(2 min. walking, nodding )
(3 min. exercising, running on spot)

full face mask – 5 min. in 1000 ppm of isoamyl acetate

II – SILICA DUST

| | Airflow | Relative Humidity & Temperature | Test Challenge | Results (unretained material) |
|---|---|---|---|---|
| Air purifying | 90 min. at 32 l/min. | | 50–60 mg/m$^3$ of flint (99+% must pass through 270 mesh sieve) | not exceed 1.5 mg |
| Powered air purifying with tight fitting facepiece | 4 hours at not less than 115 l/min. | 20–80%  25°C | Particle size distribution – (geometric mean) 0.4–0.6 micrometer | not exceed 14.4 mg |
| Powered air purifying with loose fitting hood or helmet | 4 hours at not less than 170 l/min. | | | not exceed 21.3 mg |

Table 2.1  *(continued)*

III – LEAD FUME

| | Airflow | Relative Humidity & Temperature | Test Challenge | Results (unretained material) |
|---|---|---|---|---|
| Air purifying | 90 min. at 32 l/min. | | | not exceed 1.5 mg |
| Powered air purifying with tight fitting facepiece | 4 hours at not less than 115 l/min. | 20–80% 25°C | 15–20 mg/m³ freshly generated lead oxide fume | not exceed 4.2 mg |
| Powered air purifying with loose fitting hood or helmet | 4 hours at not less than 170 l/min. | | | not exceed 6.2 mg |

IV – SILICA MIST

| | Airflow | Relative Humidity & Temperature | Test Challenge | Results (unretained material) |
|---|---|---|---|---|
| Air purifying | 90 min. at 32 l/min. | | | not exceed 2.5 mg |
| Powered air purifying with tight fitting facepiece | 4 hours at not less than 115 l/min. | 25°C | Mist produced by spraying aqueous suspension of flint (99+% of flint passes through 270 mesh sieve) | not exceed 6.9 mg |
| Powered air purifying with loose fitting hood or helmet | 4 hours at not less than 170 l/min. | | | not exceed 10.2 mg |

V - <u>PRESSURE DROP</u>

Measure before and after tests at 85 l/min.

Maximum Resistance
(mm. water column height)

| | Initial Inhalation | Final Inhalation | Exhalation |
|---|---|---|---|
| Dust, mist, fume with single use filter | 30 | 50 | 20 |
| Dust, mist, fume with reusable filter | 20 | 40 | 20 |
| Asbestos dust, mist | 18 | 25 | 15 |
| Single use | 12 | 15 | 15 |

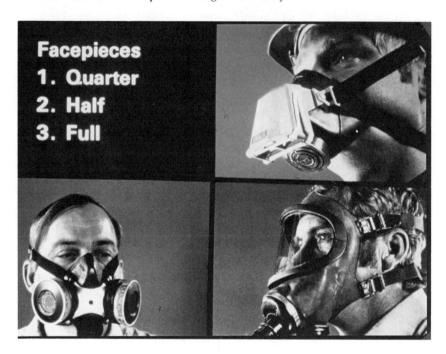

**Figure 2.6**  Different categories of mechanical-filter respirators: quarter-face *(top right);* half-face *(bottom left);* full-face *(bottom right).*

2.  They provide no protection against gases or vapors.
3.  There is a pressure drop through the filter medium; therefore, there is some breathing resistance. As the medium loads up this resistance increases; thus, people with respiratory problems should ensure that they are capable of wearing this type of respirator.

## Chemical-Cartridge Respirators

Chemical-cartridge respirators are vapor and gas-removing, using a cartridge attached to the facepiece containing chemicals to trap or react with specific vapors or gases, and remove them from the air breathed (Figure 2.7). The filtering medium is commonly activated carbon which primarily removes organic vapors. Activated carbon can also be impregnated with other substances to make it more selective against specific gases and vapors. For example, iodine is added to absorb mercury vapors; metallic oxides for acid gases; and salts of metals are added to remove ammonia.

As with mechanical-filter respirators, there are a number of factors which influence the service-life of a chemical-cartridge respirator. They are: breathing rate, humidity, contaminant concentration, temperature, etc. All

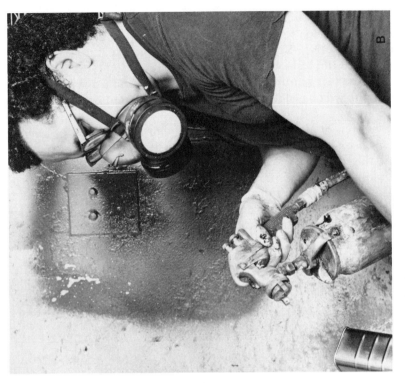

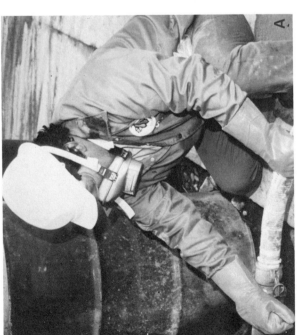

**Figure 2.7** Chemical-cartridge respirators: A. Dual cartridge—Wilson 1200 Series Respirator (courtesy of Safety Supply Canada); B. Disposable—3M Brand Ammonia Respirator #8725 (courtesy of 3M Canada).

of these factors make it very difficult to give a general statement as to how long a specific gas/vapor respirator will last.

In order to be NIOSH-approved a gas/vapor respirator must pass a number of service-life tests which are outlined in 30CFR11.162-8. Table 2.2 summarizes these test requirements. One of the test requirements is a *minimum service-life* which is determined when the permitted penetration value is detected.

Gary Nelson et al published a series of eight articles in the *American Industrial Hygiene Association Journal* between 1972 and 1976 titled, "Respirator Cartridge Efficiency Studies," and determined that humidity, organic vapor volatility, concentration, carbon weight, contaminant molecular weight and breathing rate all play a role in influencing cartridge service-life [4-11]. They concluded that solvent type, flow rate, solvent concentrations and relative humidity were the four major influencing factors in determining

Table 2.2  Summary of NIOSH test requirements for chemical cartridge respirators

| | | Test Atmosphere | | | | |
| | | Gas or Vapour | Concentration (ppm) | Flow rate (lpm) | Penetration (ppm) | Min. life (min) |
| Cartridge | Test Condition | | | | | |
|---|---|---|---|---|---|---|
| Ammonia ........... | As received ... | $NH_3$ | 1000 | 64 | 50 | 50 |
| Ammonia ........... | Equilibrated .. | $NH_3$ | 1000 | 32 | 50 | 50 |
| Chlorine .......... | As received ... | $Cl_2$ | 500 | 64 | 5 | 35 |
| Chlorine .......... | Equilibrated .. | $Cl_2$ | 500 | 32 | 5 | 35 |
| Hydrogen Chloride .. | As received ... | HCl | 500 | 64 | 5 | 50 |
| Hydrogen Chloride .. | Equilibrated .. | HCl | 500 | 32 | 5 | 50 |
| Methyl amine ....... | As received ... | $CH_3NH_3$ | 1000 | 64 | 10 | 25 |
| Methyl amine ....... | Equilibrated .. | $CH_3NH_3$ | 1000 | 32 | 10 | 25 |
| Organic vapours .... | As received ... | $CCl_4$ | 1000 | 64 | 5 | 50 |
| Organic vapours .... | Equilibrated .. | $CCl_4$ | 1000 | 32 | 3 | 50 |
| Sulfur dioxide ..... | As received ... | $SO_3$ | 500 | 64 | 5 | 30 |
| Sulfur dioxide ..... | Equilibrated .. | $SO_3$ | 500 | 32 | 5 | 30 |

MAXIMUM RESISTANCE
(mm water-column height)

| Type of chemical cartridge respirator | Inhalation | | Exhalation |
| | Initial | Final | |
|---|---|---|---|
| For gases, vapours, or gases and vapours ................... | 40 | 45 | 20 |
| For gases, vapours, or gases and vapours, and dusts, fumes, and mists .................... | 50 | 70 | 20 |
| For gases, vapours, or gases and vapours, and mists of paints, lacquers, and enamels ......... | 50 | 70 | 20 |

cartridge service life. We refer you to their paper for specific details and results of their experiments, but their results can be summarized as follows:

1. Each organic vapor has different adsorption characteristics on carbon. In general it is felt that the higher the volatility of the vapor, the less efficiently it adsorbs into the carbon.
2. The more carbon available the longer the service-life is. Doubling the amount of carbon will generally double the service-life.
3. Breakthrough time is inversely proportional to the flow-rate. That is, halving the flow rate will double the service-life.
4. The service-life is inversely proportional to the log of the concentration.
5. Service-life is shorter if the relative humidity is greater than 65%. If the humidity is less than 50% the service-life is not noticeably affected.

It is not an easy matter to determine the actual service-life of a gas/vapor respirator because of all the variables that have influence. The best policy is to replace the respirator or cartridge when an odor or taste is detected (Table 2.3, odor thresholds); it becomes hard to breath through; or the cartridge or respirator is damaged [12]. The *American Industrial Hygiene Association Journal* published in 1976 an equation which can be used to calculate the predicted service-life of a chemical cartridge at a given exposure concentration [11]. This equation is as follows:

$$t_{10\%} = \frac{2.4 \times 10^6 \, W_c \, (a + bt)}{c^{2/3} \, MQ}$$

where:  $t_{10\%}$ = service-time (minutes) of a cartridge to 10% chemical breakthrough

$W_c$ = weight of cartridge (grams)

a,b = solvent coefficients

t = boiling point of the chemical (°C)

c = airborne concentration of the chemical (ppm)

M = molecular weight of the chemical

Q = average breathing rate for moderate work (30 liters/minute)

Thus, if the average concentration of the gas or vapor in the workplace is known, this equation can be used to predict when respirator cartridges should be changed. A safety factor should be built in and it is recommended that a 50% safety factor be applied when predicting the service-life of a chemical-cartridge respirator. The final judgment of the service-life should be with the wearer.

The effectiveness of gas and vapor respirators depends on their ability to remove chemical molecules from the air stream. Molecules of gas and vapor are much smaller than aerosol particles and are not removed by fiber

Table 2.3   Odor threshold for selected contaminants

| COMPOUND | ODOUR THRESHOLD (ppm/v) | COMPOUND | ODOUR THRESHOLD (ppm/v) |
|---|---|---|---|
| Acetaldehyde | 0.031 - 0.21 | Apiol | 0.0063 |
| Acetic acid | 1.0 - 24 | Benzene | 4.68 - 31.0 |
| Acetone | 40.0 - 100.0 | Benzyl chloride | 0.04 |
| Acetophenone | 0.17 - 17.0 | Benzyl mercaptan | 0.0026 |
| Acrolein | $1.1 \times 10^{-5}$ - 1.5 | Benzyl sulphide | 0.002 - 0.006 |
| Acrylonitrile | 19.0 - 21.4 | Bromine | 0.047 - 1.0 |
| Allyl alcohol | 0.017 - 1.4 | Bromoacetone | 0.090 |
| Allyl amine | 6.3 | Butadiene | 0.16 - 0.45 |
| Allyl chloride | $1.5 \times 10^{-4}$ - 0.47 | i-Butane | 1.2 |
| Allyl isocyanide | 0.018 | n-Butanol | 5.0 - 11.0 |
| Allyl isothiocyanide | 0.008 - 0.15 | s-Butanol | 43.0 |
| Allyl mercaptan | $5 \times 10^{-5}$ - 0.004 | t-Butanol | 73.0 |
| Allyl sulphide | $1.4 \times 10^{-4}$ | 2-Butanone | 2 - 80 |
| Ammonia | 34 - 55 | Butyl acetate | 20.0 |
| n-Amyl acetate | 0.005 - 0.08 | Butyl formate | 17.0 |
| Amyl alcohol | 0.12 - 35.0 | Butyl mercaptan | 0.006 |
| Amylene | 0.0022 - 2.1 | Butyl sulphide | 0.015 |
| i - Amyl mercaptan | 0.0043 | Butyric acid | $5.6 \times 10^{-4}$ - 0.4 |
| | | Camphor | 1.2 - 1.6 |
| Amyl sulphide | 0.003 | Carbon disulphide | 0.0081 - 0.02 |
| Anethole | 0.003 | | |
| | | Carbon monoxide | Odourless |
| Aniline | 1.0 - 70.0 | | |

Table 2.3   *(continued)*

| COMPOUND | ODOUR THRESHOLD (ppm/v) | COMPOUND | ODOUR THRESHOLD (ppm/v) |
|---|---|---|---|
| Carbon tetrachloride | 21.0 - 200.0 | Dimethyl sulphide | 0.02 |
| Chloral | 0.047 | Dioxane | 0.8 - 170.0 |
| Chlorine | 0.01 - 0.3 | Diphenyl-chlorarsine | 0.03 |
| Chlorine dioxide | 0.1 | | |
| Chlorobenzene | 0.21 - 94.0 | Diphenyl-cyanoarsine | 0.3 |
| Chloroform | 200.0 | Diphenylether | 0.1 |
| m-Cresol | 0.01 - 0.68 | Diphenyl sulphide | 0.0021-0.0047 |
| o-Cresol | 0.09 - 0.68 | | |
| Crotonaldehyde | 0.035 - 1.6 | Diphosgene | 1.2 |
| Cyclohexane | 0.41 | Dithioethylene glycol | 0.031 |
| o-Dichloro-benzene | 50 | Dodecanol | 0.0064 |
| 1,1-Dichloro-ethane | 120 | Ethane | 89.9 - 150.0 |
| | | 1,2-Ethanedithiol | 0.0031-0.0042 |
| 1,2-Dichloro-propane | 50 | Ethanol | 0.1 - 5100 |
| Diethylamine | 0.006 - 30.0 | Ethyl acetate | 0.056 |
| Diethyl selenide | $1.4 \times 10^{-4}$ | Ethyl acrylate | 0.00047 |
| Diethyl sulphide | 0.004 | Ethyl butyrate | 0.0082 - 0.015 |
| | | Ethyl decanoate | 0.00017 |
| Dimethyl acetamide | 46.8 | Ethyl dichloroarsine | 1.4 |
| Dimethyl-formamide | 100.0 | Ethyl ether | 0.33 |
| 1,1-Dimethyl hydrazine | 6.0 | Ethyl glycol | 25 |

Table 2.3    *(continued)*

| COMPOUND | ODOUR THRESHOLD (ppm/v) | COMPOUND | ODOUR THRESHOLD (ppm/v) |
|---|---|---|---|
| Ethyl mercaptan | $1.9 \times 10^{-4}$ – $5.1 \times 10^{-4}$ | Hydrogen chloride | 10.0 |
| Ethyl metacrylate | 0.0067 | Hydrogen sulphide | 0.0081 – 0.12 |
| Ethyl pelargonate | 0.0014 | Iodoform | $5.0 \times 10^{-4}$ |
| Ethyl selenide | 0.0012 | Light gasoline | 800.0 |
| Ethyl selenomer-captan | $3 \times 10^{-4}$ – $12 \times 10^{-3}$ | Menthol | 1.5 |
|  |  | 2-Mercapto-ethanol | 0.64 |
| Ethyl sulphide | $6.0 \times 10^{-4}$ – 0.002 | Mesitylene | 0.027 |
| Ethyl i-valerate | 0.12 | Methanol | 4.3 – 5900 |
| Ethyl n-valerate | 0.060 | Methoxynaphtha-lene | $1.2 \times 10^{-4}$ |
| Ethylene | $4.0 \times 10^{-3}$ – 260 | Methyl acetate | 200.0 |
| Ethylene bromide | 25.0 | Methyl amine | 0.02 – 3.3 |
| Ethylene glycol | 0.080 | 2-Methyl-2-butanol | 2.3 |
| Ethylene oxide | 260 – 700 | Methyl n-Butynate | 0.0026 |
| Ethylene undecanoate | $5.4 \times 10^{-4}$ | Methyl chloride | 10.0 |
| Eugenol | 0.0046 | Methyl dichloro arsine | 0.11 |
| Formaldehyde | 0.98 – 49.9 | Methyl ehtyl pyridine | 0.05 |
| Formic acid | 0.025 – 21.0 | Methyl formate | 2000 |
| n-Heptane | 22.0 | Methyl glycol | 60.0 |
| Hexanol | 0.0050 – 5.2 |  |  |
| Hydrazine | 3.0 | Methyl isobutyl ketone | 0.1 – 3.0 |
| Hydrocyanic acid | $2.7 \times 10^{-4}$ – 0.001 |  |  |

Table 2.3   *(continued)*

| COMPOUND | ODOUR THRESHOLD (ppm/v) | COMPOUND | ODOUR THRESHOLD (ppm/v) |
|---|---|---|---|
| Methyl mercaptan | 0.041 | n-Pentane | 2.2 |
| Methyl metacrylate | 0.051 - 0.21 | Pentanol | 0.0065 - 1.0 |
| | | Pentanone | 8.0 - 70 |
| 2-Methyl propane | 0.57 | i-Pentyl acetate | 0.0028 |
| Methyl salicylate | 0.006 | n-Pentyl acetate | $9.0 \times 10^{-4}$ |
| Methyl sulphide | 0.00015 - 0.012 | Propyl mercaptan | 0.0016 |
| Methyl thiocyanate | 0.25 | Propyl sulphide | 0.011 |
| | | Pyridine | 0.03 - 0.82 |
| Methyl vinyl pyridine | 0.04 | Styrene | 0.047 - 37 |
| Methylene chloride | 150 - 210 | Sulphur dioxide | 0.47 - 3.0 |
| Musk (synthetic) | $4.0 \times 10^{-7}$ - 0.004 | Tetrachloro-ethylene | 4.6 - 50 |
| | | Tetrahydrofuran | 30 |
| Naphthalene | 0.027 - 6.8 | Toluene | 1.7 - 40 |
| 2-Naphthol | 1.3 | Toluene-2,4 diisocyanite | 2.1 |
| Nitric oxide | 1.0 | | |
| Nitrobenzene | 0.0047 - 1.9 | Trichloro-ethylene | 21.0 - 400 |
| n-Octane | 150 | Trimethylamine | $2.1 \times 10^{-4}$ -1.7 |
| Octanoic acid | 0.0014 - 35.0 | Valeric acid | $6.0 \times 10^{4}$ |
| 1-Octanol | 0.0021 - 0.1 | Vanillin | $3.2 \times 10^{-8}$ - 0.68 |
| 2-Octanol | 0.0026 | o-Xylene | 20 |
| Oenanthic acid | 0.015 | m-Xylene | 3.7 |
| Ozone | 0.02 | p-Xylene | 0.49 |
| Pelargonic acid | $8.6 \times 10^{-4}$ - 5.0 | Xylidene | 0.0048 |

filters. It is necessary to bring the molecules in contact with the sorbent material which reacts with the contaminant. The reaction may be one of chemical combining (KOH + HCl) or one of physical chemistry force (organic vapor and charcoal). Absorption and adsorption both may occur. Absorption is penetration; adsorption is adherence.

The chemical reaction, absorption or adsorption process, is 100% efficient until the sorbent's capacity to filter out the contaminant is exhausted. At that time the contaminant will pass completely through the sorbent material and into the facepiece. The *breakthrough* of the gas or vapor is generally the only way the wearer knows that the respirator is used up. Therefore, chemical-cartridge respirators can only be used against contaminants when good warning properties are employed, that is, those that can be tasted or smelled at concentrations which are not toxic.

When particulates, gases and vapors are present in the same environment, particulate prefitters can be placed in front of the chemical cartridge, thus providing a combination particulate/gas and vapor respirator (Figure 2.8).

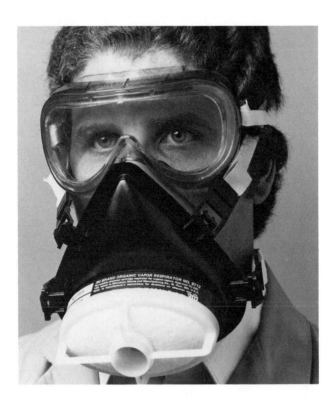

**Figure 2.8** Combination particulate/vapor respirator: 3M Brand Organic Vapor Respirator #8712 with Prefilter #8733 (courtesy of 3M Canada).

As with the mechanical-filter respirator, the chemical-cartridge respirator is available as cartridge-type or disposable. Also they are available in quarter, half and full-face designs.

There are a number of limitations to the use of chemical-cartridge respirators which one must be aware of when selecting the proper respiratory protection. These limitations are:

1.  They do not supply oxygen and thus cannot be worn in oxygen-deficient atmospheres.
2.  These respirators are designed for protection against specific gases or vapors. One must make sure that he reads the label carefully and understands what the cartridge is designed for. A cartridge designed for acid gases may not provide adequate protection against organic vapors.
3.  These respirators can be used for protection against contaminants with good warning properties (smell, taste, irritation). The respirator works at 100% efficiency until the capacity of the sorbent is reached, then the contaminant passes through the sorbent material and is inhaled by the wearer. Thus there must be a warning system that alerts the wearer that the chemical cartridge is used up, and that the wearer can be exposed to the hazardous material.
4.  They must not be used in atmospheres immediately dangerous to life or health, except when an escape is necessary.
5.  These respirators must be protected from the atmosphere while in storage because they tend to pick up water vapor from the air. This may reduce or increase the effectiveness of the sorbent. Also the sorbent will continue to pick up the contaminant even if it is left in the work environment and it is not being worn. This will reduce the useful life of the respirator.

**Gas Masks**

The third class of air-purifying respirators is the gas mask. Gas masks are designed to protect against slightly higher concentrations of organic vapors or gases, alkaline gases, acid gases, pesticides, paint vapors and mists, radioactive particulates, dust, mists, fumes and certain combinations of these materials. Nearly all gas masks have a full facepiece (Figure 2.9).

The basic difference between a full-facepiece chemical-cartridge respirator and a gas mask is the volume of sorbent contained within. The volume of sorbent contained in a canister is in the order of 2 to 10 times that contained in a cartridge.

There are essentially two versions of gas masks, the first one being the front or back-mounted gas mask. Generally with this version, a super-size or industrial-size canister is fastened to the user's body, either front or back, and a breathing tube connects the canister to the facepiece inlet. The volume

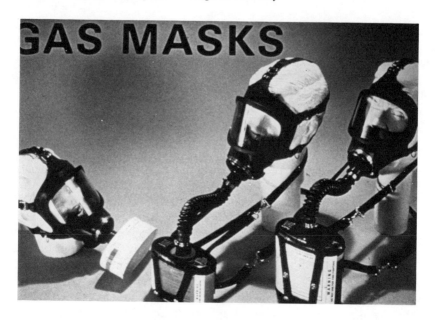

**Figure 2.9**  Gas masks.

of sorbent contained in the canister is in the range of 1000–2000 cm³. The inhalation valve is also contained in the canister and not in the facepiece as in chemical-cartridge respirators.

The super-size canister is somewhat larger than the industrial-size canister and has approximately twice the useful time of the industrial-size canister. Both canister sizes have various types that are specific for the gas and/ or vapor contaminant, and are also labeled with an expiration date and may have a window indicator to assist in evaluating the remaining service-life. The canisters are also color-coded as per the American National Standard, ANSI K.13.1. Again, this color code should not be relied on solely, and the user should always read the label and other pertinent information supplied with the equipment.

The second version of gas mask is the chin-style. Chin-style gas masks typically have a medium-sized canister rigidly attached to a full facepiece. The volume of sorbent contained in the canister is normally in the range of 250-500 cm³. The useful lifetime is less than that of a front or back-mounted canister but greater than that of chemical cartridges, owing to the smaller sorbent volume.

Canister-type gas masks are designed for use in an atmosphere with known gas concentrations not exceeding 2% by volume (20,000 ppm.) or as indicated on the canister label. They are generally available for protection against organic vapors, acids, gases or ammonia.

As with the previous two types of air-purifying respirators, gas masks do not provide protection against oxygen deficiency.

## Powered Air-Purifying Respirators

The powered air-purifying respirator uses a blower to pass contaminated air through a filtering medium (Figure 2.10). It may be used for particulate, vapors or gases, or a combination of these. The filter medium may be located in a belt-mount holder (Figure 2.11), or in the headpiece (Figure 2.12). Air is passed through the filter by use of a blower and delivered to a facepiece or head cover (Figure 2.13). This type of air-purifying respirator has a distinct advantage because it puts the facepiece or headpiece under positive pressure with respect to the outside contaminated atmosphere, so that any leakage is outward from the facepiece. The limitations of these respirators are as follows:

1. These do not supply oxygen, therefore, they cannot be worn in oxygen-deficient atmospheres.
2. The type and degree of protection depends on the air-purifying element whose protection level and useful service-time depend, in turn, on its

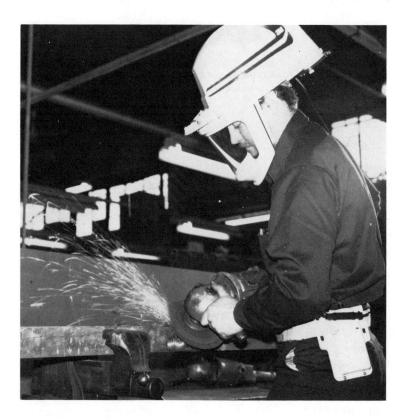

**Figure 2.10** Powered air-purifying respirator: 3M Brand Airhat (courtesy of 3M Canada).

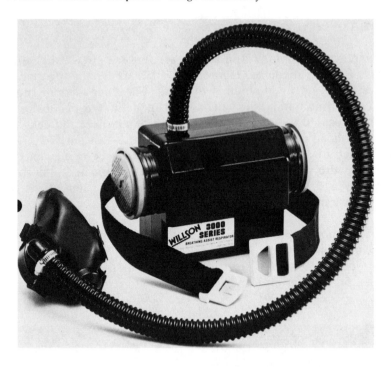

**Figure 2.11**  Belt-mounted air-purifying respirator: Wilson 3000 Series Breathing Assist Respirator (courtesy of Safety Supply Canada).

material, size, and shape, and also on the nature and concentration of the contaminant.

## ATMOSPHERE-SUPPLYING RESPIRATORS

The atmosphere-supplying class of respirators differ from the air-purifying class in that air is provided from a source independent of the surrounding atmosphere instead of purifying the atmosphere. Thus, the user is breathing within a system, which admits no outside air. There are essentially three kinds of atmosphere-supplying respirators:

1.  Self-contained breathing apparatus (SCBA), where the user carries a supply of respirable air (Figure 2.14).
2.  Supplied air-line where the user is supplied with respirable air through a hose (Figure 2.15).
3.  Combination SCBA and supplied air-line.

In all cases the air supply must conform, or meet, the requirements of the Compressed Gas Association Specification 67.1 (ANSI Z86.1973) for

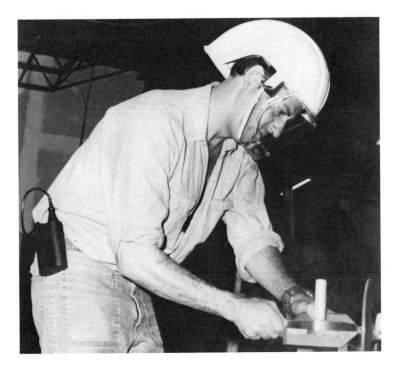

**Figure 2.12** Power air-purifying respirator: filter located in the head piece. Racal Airstream (courtesy of Safety Supply Canada).

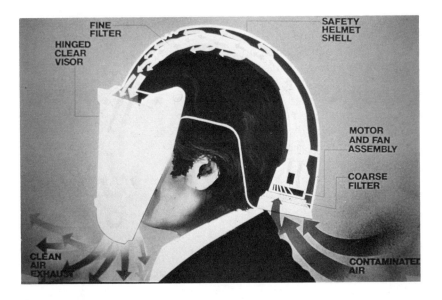

**Figure 2.13** Operation of powered air-purifying respirator.

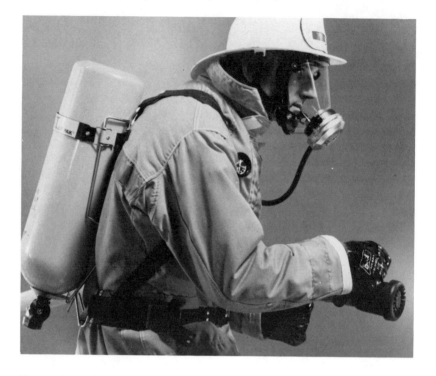

**Figure 2.14**   Self-contained breathing apparatus (courtesy of Safety Supply Canada).

Type 1, Class D gaseous air. This means that the carbon monoxide level must not exceed 20 ppm., carbon dioxide must not exceed 1000 ppm., and condensed hydrocarbons must not exceed 5 mg./m.$^3$.

There are many different types of self-contained breathing apparati. These different types may be differentiated in two ways: by the method by which air is supplied and by the way in which the air supply is regulated.

There are essentially two ways in which air can be supplied; the first way is the rebreathing type or closed-circuit SCBA. In this type of system the air is rebreathed after the exhaled carbon dioxide has been removed and the oxygen content restored by a compressed oxygen source or an oxygen-generating substance. These devices are designed primarily for 1- to 4-hour use in oxygen-deficient atmospheres, and once initiated, normally cannot be turned off. In one type of closed-circuit device, the exhaled air passes through a granular solid absorbent that removes the carbon dioxide, thus reducing the flow back into the breathing bag. The bag collapses, thus opening the admission valve to admit more pure oxygen that reinflates the bag. The oxygen, again, is supplied from a compressed oxygen or an oxygen-generating substance, such as potassium superoxide.

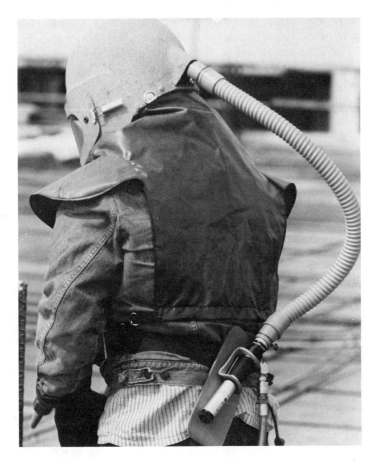

**Figure 2.15**  Supplied air-line respirator (courtesy of 3M Canada).

Another type of closed-circuit system is the oxygen-generating self-contained apparatus. This system functions differently from the compressed oxygen cylinder type because there are no mechanical operating components. This unit works on the lung-governing principle wherein the wearers of the apparatus, by their own breathing, regulate the oxygen supply automatically and provide the exact amount required. The oxygen-generating solid is usually potassium superoxide, $KO_2$. The $H_2O$ and $CO_2$ in the exhaled breath react with the $KO_2$ to release $O_2$. This device is front mounted and consists of a hermetically sealed canister containing the chemical, a housing into which the canister is inserted, a breathing bag, breathing tubes, facepiece and harness assembly.

The second method in which air can be supplied is via an air cylinder, which is common in the open-circuit SCBA. An open-circuit SCBA exhausts the exhaled air to the atmosphere instead of recirculating it. A tank of high-pressure compressed air, normally carried on the back, supplies air to a two-stage regulator that reduces the pressure for delivery to the facepiece. The service-life of the open circuit SCBA is normally shorter than a closed-circuit system, since it has to provide the total breathing requirements and not just the oxygen requirements for recirculation of air. Most open-circuit devices have a service life of 30 minutes, and 15 minutes or less for special circumstances, with smaller air cylinders.

As previously mentioned, in addition to the method by which air is supplied, many different types of SCBA can also be differentiated by the way in which the air supply is regulated. Air is regulated to the facepiece by two different modes; the first being demand. In the demand-type regulator, air at approximately 200° PSI is supplied to the admission valve via a two-stage regulator which reduces the pressure to approximately 50–100 PSI. The admission valve is activated upon inhalation which creates negative pressure in the facepiece, which in turn contracts a diaphragm causing the admission valve to open and allow air into the facepiece. The admission valve remains closed as long as positive pressure is maintained in the facepiece. In other words, air flows into the facepiece only on "demand" by the wearer, hence the name.

The second type is called pressure-demand. A pressure-demand regulator is very similar to the demand-type except for a spring between the diaphragm and the outside case of the regulator. This spring tends to hold the admission valve slightly open, theoretically allowing continual airflow into the facepiece. This would be true except that all pressure-demand devices have a special exhalation valve that maintains about 1.5–3 inches of water positive-back pressure in the facepiece, and opens only when the pressure exceeds that value. This combination of modified regulator and special exhalation valve maintains positive pressure in the facepiece at all times, and the regulator still supplies additional air on demand. The designed air flowrate for demand and pressure-demand regulators is approximately 350–400 LPM.

It should be noted here that a facepiece whose exhalation valve is designed for demand operation cannot be used with a pressure-demand regulator, since air will flow continuously and quickly exhaust the air supply. However, contrary to this, some open-circuit SCBAs are designed with the capability of switching from demand to pressure-demand.

All SCBAs may be used in oxygen-deficient atmospheres. However, only full-facepiece positive-pressure units (i.e., pressure-demand) should be used in IDLH environments. Half-mask demand SCBA units are believed to provide no more protection against toxic substances than most air-purifying devices. All SCBA equipment must also have a functioning remaining service-life indicator or warning device that signals when only 20-25% of service-time remains.

The second kind of atmosphere-supplying respirator is the supplied air-line. Supplied air-line respirators use a central source of breathing air that is delivered to the wearer through an air-supply line or hose (Figure 2.16). The hose-length varies from 25 to 300 feet and the maximum-inlet operating pressure must not exceed 125 PSIG, at the point where the hose attaches to the air supply.

The air-line respirators may consist of a half-mask, full facepiece, hood or helmet, or as a complete suit in certain applications. Full-suit air-line respirators are used against substances that irritate, corrode or penetrate through the skin, and they also provide breathing air. Designs for abrasive blasting are also available, which provide protection against impact and abrasion from rebounding material.

Air-line respirators are available in demand, pressure-demand and continuous-flow configurations. A demand or pressure-demand air-line respirator is very similar to a demand or pressure-demand open-circuit SCBA, except that the air is supplied through a small-diameter hose from a stationary source of compressed air rather than from a portable high-pressure hose. Regulators for air-line respirators also have only single-stage reduction as opposed to two-stage, because the air pressure is limited to 125 PSI.

Continuous-flow air-line respirators maintain air flow at all times, rather than only on demand. In place of a demand or pressure-demand regulator, an air-flow control valve or orifice partially controls the air-flow. The air-flow must be at least 4 CFM to a facepiece or 6 CFM to a helmet or hood.

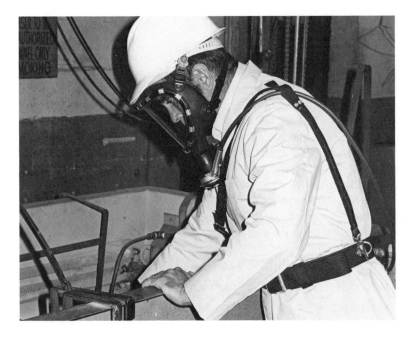

**Figure 2.16** Supplied air-line respirator (courtesy of Safety Supply Canada).

The stationary source of compressed air could be from a compressed air cylinder, a compressor or purified, compressed plant air. Caution should be maintained to ensure that the breathing air is free of unwanted contaminants and meets the requirements of Compressed Gas Association Specification 67.1 (ANSI Z86.1973) for Type 1, Class D gaseous air.

Supplied-air-line respirators provide a high degree of protection, but their use is limited to atmospheres not immediately dangerous to life and health, for the wearer is totally dependent upon the integrity of the air-supply hose and he must be able to escape from the contaminated area without endangering his life.

The last kind of an atmosphere-supplying respirator is the combination SCBA and supplied air-line. This type is essentially the same as the air-line respirator, with an added compressed-air cylinder that may be carried on one's back or at one's side in a sling. Combination units may consist of a half-mask or full facepiece and operate in the demand or pressure-demand mode.

Combination units are generally used for emergency entry into and escape from atmospheres immediately dangerous to life and health. The self-contained part of the device is used only when the air-line part fails and the wearer must escape, or when it may be necessary to disconnect the air-line temporarily while changing locations. A combination air-line and SCBA may also be used for emergency entry into a hazardous atmosphere to connect to an air-line, if the SCBA is classified for service of 15 minutes or longer and not more than 20% of the air supply's rated capacity is used during entry.

In summary, the basic purpose of a respirator is to protect the respiratory system from harmful airborne contaminants. It does this by removing—through mechanical filtration, chemical reaction, adsorption or absorption—the contaminant from the air, or by supplying an independent source of breathable air. Selection of the proper type of respirator will provide workers with the necessary protection they require. There are limitations to the usage of all types of respirators and these must be understood. This chapter has summarized the different types of respirators available on the market today and their corresponding limitations. More detailed information on specific respirators or types of respirators can be obtained from respirator manufacturers. Manufacturers or distributors of NIOSH/MSHA approved respiratory devices include:

Ace Enterprises, 820 Northwest 144th St., Miami, FL 33168.

Acme Automotive Finishes, 101 Prospect Avenue, Cleveland, OH 44115.

American Optical Corp., Safety Products Div., 100 Canal St., Putnam, CT 06260.

Anderson Manufacturing Co., 1014 Fox Chase Road, Rockledge, PA 19111.

Binks Manufacturing Co., 9201 W. Belmont Ave., Franklin Park, IL 60131.

BioMarine Industries, Inc., 45 Great Valley Center, Malvern, PA 19355.

Bowen Tools Inc., P.O. Box 3186, Houston, TX 77001.

E.D. Bullard Co., 2680 Bridgeway, Sausalito, CA 94965.

Cesco Safety Products, Parmelee Industries, Inc., P.O. Box 1237, Kansas City, MO 64141.

Clemco Industries, 2177 Jerrold Avenue, San Francisco, CA 94124.

Clemtex Ltd., 248 McCarthy Drive, Houston, TX 77020.

H.S. Cover Co., 107 East Alexander Street, Buchanan, MI 49107.

DeVilbiss Company, 300 Phillips Avenue, P.O. Box 913, Toledo, OH 43692.

Dragerwerk, AG, D-24 Luebeck 1, Postfach 1339, Germany.

Eastern Safety Equipment Co., 45-17 Pearson St., Long Island City, NY 11101.

Empire Abrasive Equipment Corp., 9990 Gantry Road, Philadelphia, PA 19115.

Encon Manufacturing Co., 4914 Dickson St., Houston, TX 77007.

Fiber-Metal, P.O. Box 248, Concordville, PA 19331.

Glendale Optical Co., 130 Crossways Park Drive, Woodbury, NY 11797.

Globe Safety Products, Inc., 125 Sunrise Place, Dayton, OH 45407.

Kelco Sales & Engineering Co., P.O. Box 422, Norwalk, CA 90650.

Key Houston, Inc., 13911 Atlanta Blvd., Jacksonville, FL 32225.

Lear Siegler, Inc., 714 North Brookhurst St., Anaheim, CA 92803.

Mine Safety Appliances Co., 600 Penn Center Blvd., Pittsburgh, PA 15235.

Northcott Products Company, 1826 West Diverse Parkway, Chicago, IL 60614.

Norton Safety Products, 2000 Plainfield Pike, Cranston, RI 02920.

Pauli & Griffin, 137 Utah Avenue, South San Francisco, CA 94080.

Pulmosan Safety Equipment Corp., 30–48 Linden Place, Flushing, NY 11354.

Racal Airstream Inc., 5 Research Place, Rockville, MD 20850.

Robertshaw Controls Co., 333 North Euclid Way, Anaheim, CA 92803.

Safe-Tex, Toronto, Ontario, Canada.

Schmidt Manufacturing Inc., Houston, TX.

Scott Aviation, Division of ATO, Inc., Lancaster, NY 14086.

Sellstrom Manufacturing Co., 59 E. Van Buren Street, Chicago, IL 60605.

Siebe Gorman, Ltd., Chessington Surrey, England.

Stewart-Warner, Chicago, IL 60614.

Survivair, Division of U.S. Divers Co., 3323 W. Warner Ave., Santa Ana, CA 92702.

Titan Abrasive Systems, Inc., P.O. Box 3, Furlong, PA 18925.

3M Company, 3M Center, St. Paul, MN 55101.

U.S. Safety Service, Parmelee Industries, Inc., P.O. Box 1237, Kansas City, MO 64141.

Willson Products Division, INCO, P.O. Box 1733, Reading, PA 19603.

The source for this listing is AIHA, Respiratory Protection—A Manual and Guideline [13].

## REFERENCES

1.  Japuntich, D.A., "Respiratory Particulate Filtration," *Journal of the International Society of Respiratory Protection,* 2(1), 1984:137–168.
2.  Van Turnhout, J., Van Bochove, C., and van Veldhuizen, G.J., "Electret fibres for high-efficiency filtration of polluted gases," *Staub-Reinhold Luft,* 36, 1976:36–39.
3.  Federal Register Vol. 37, No. 59, Title 30, Pg. 6243–6271.
4.  Ruch, W.E., Nelson, G.O., Lindeken, C.L., Johnson, R.E., and Hodgkins, D.J., "Respirator Cartridge Efficiency Studies: I. Experimental Design," *American Industrial Hygiene Association Journal* 33:105 (1972).
5.  Nelson, G.O. and Hodgkins, D.J.: "Respirator Cartridge Efficiency Studies: II. Preparation of Test Atmospheres," *American Industrial Hygiene Association Journal* 33:110 (1972).
6.  Nelson, G.O., Johnson, R.E., Lindeken, C.L., and Taylor, R.D.: "Respirator Cartridge Efficiency Studies: III. A Mechanical Breathing Machine to Simulate Human Respiration," *American Industrial Hygiene Association Journal* 33:745 (1972).
7.  Nelson, G.O. and Harder, C.A.: "Respirator Cartridge Efficiency Studies: IV. Effects of Steady State and Pulsating Flow," *American Industrial Hygiene Association Journal* 33:391 (1974).
8.  Nelson, G.O. and Harder, C.A.: "Respirator Cartridge Efficiency Studies: V. Effects of Solvent Vapor," *American Industrial Hygiene Association Journal* 33:391 (1974).
9.  Nelson, G.O., Harder, C.A., and Bigler, B.E.: "Respirator Cartridge Efficiency Studies: VI. Effect of Concentration," *Lawrence Livermore Laboratory, Report* UCRL-76184 (Nov. 1974).
10. Nelson, G.O., Correia, A.M., and Harder, C.A.: "Respirator Cartridge Efficiency Studies: VII. Effect of Relative Humidity and Temperature," *Lawrence Livermore Laboratory, Report* UCRL-77390 (Aug. 1975).
11. Nelson, G.O. and Correia, A.N.: "Respirator Cartridge Efficiency Studies: VIII. Summary and Conclusions," *American Industrial Hygiene Association Journal* 37:514 (1976).

12. Canadian Standards Association Standard Z94-4-M1982, "Selection, Care and Use of Respirators," Appendix 1 (1982).
13. Birkner, L.R., "Respiratory Protection: A Manual and Guideline," American Industrial Hygiene Association. Edited by B.J. Held and B.E. Held (1980).

# 3

## *Criteria for Selection and Fitting*

Before we discuss the selection and fitting of respirators, we would like to briefly summarize the regulatory requirements that govern the use of respiratory protection in the workplace. In Chapter 7 a respiratory protection program will be discussed while this chapter and Chapters 4, 5, and 6 will expand on the program elements. The key components of the respiratory protection program have come about because of regulatory requirements, so it is worthwhile for the reader to be familiar with these regulatory requirements.

The various regulatory authorities in industrialized nations appear to have accepted the fact that very low acceptable levels of exposure to airborne contaminants cannot be achieved with engineering controls alone, and hence, must be augmented by respiratory protective equipment. This realization has prompted them to set out various criteria and guidelines for testing and approving respirators. Some of these guidelines are minimum requirements for employers in order to provide an adequate respiratory protection program for employees.

Some of these minimum requirements may include:

- Written procedures for selection and use of respirators, fitting, training and cleaning;
- Pre-use and annual physical examinations to ensure that the employee is physically able to wear and work in the equipment;
- Selection and use of respirators on the basis of the hazard(s) involved;
- Development of a training program designed to train workers in the correct method of wearing and using a respirator;
- Regular, periodic cleaning, inspecting, repairing and disinfecting of used respirators.

The requirements also state that approved or accepted respirators should be used when they are available. In theory, a regulatory authority may accept a respirator evaluated by any competent authority. However, in North

America only, three organizations have been historically recognized as competent, namely, the United States National Institute for Occupational Safety and Health (NIOSH), the United States Mine Safety and Health Administration (MSHA) and the British Standards Institute (BSI).

## HISTORY OF APPROVAL OF RESPIRATORS IN THE UNITED STATES

The Bureau of Mines in 1919 brought out the first approval schedule. This included:

SCHEDULE:   13.   Self-Contained Breathing Apparatus (SCBA)
            14.   Gas Mask (full-face mask)
            19.   Air-Line Respirators
            21.   Dust, Fume and Mist Respirators (D.F.M.)
            23.   New Emergency Organic Vapor Respirators, O.V.

As the schedules were revised over the years, alphabets were included with the numbers, e.g., 13A, 13B, etc.

There were two problems with this scheduling system:
1.  There were no provisions for de-certification, e.g., a CHEMOX Oxygen Breathing Apparatus purchased under Schedule 13, in 1919, would still be approved today, and
2.  More than half the respirators were being used above ground in nonmining operations.

NIOSH and MSHA started the present respirator-approval program in 1971 when they assumed U.S. Bureau of Mines (BOM) responsibilities. All testing for approvals is performed by NIOSH and the results are reviewed by NIOSH and MSHA who are the approval agencies. The Williams and Steiger Occupational Safety and Health Act (OSHA) was enacted in 1970. It sets forth specific legal requirements for selection, use, and maintenance of respirators, and gives guidelines for establishing a respirator program to meet these requirements. These requirements are outlined in Title 30, Code of Federal Regulation, Part II, commonly known as "Part II" [1].
Schedules and terminology have changed as follows:

Part II,   Subpart H—Self-Contained Breathing Apparatus
                      (Old Schedule 13F)
           Subpart I—Gas Masks (Schedule 14G)
           Subpart J—Supplied-Air Respirators (Schedule 19C)
           Subpart K—Dust, Fume and Mist Respirators (Schedule 21C)
           Subpart L—Chemical-Cartridge Respirators (Schedule 23C)
           Subpart M—Pesticide Respirators (Schedule 23C)

In the transition period, respirators with Bureau of Mines' approval could be used until March 30, 1974. However, grandfather clauses and extensions have allowed some Bureau of Mines' respirators to be used legally, e.g., gas masks under Schedule 14F, self-contained breathing apparatus, Schedule 13-13F (good until March 31, 1979).

Generally, it is difficult to determine if a respirator (in total) is approved unless a person is experienced. Simply put, there must be absolutely no change to the respirator, (e.g., missing parts, incorrect parts) which has passed the approval schedule, or else that respirator is not approved. The respirator(s) in question must be checked against manufacturers' literature and the *NIOSH Certified Equipment List* which is updated every year [2].

After submission by manufacturers, respirators which are in the process of being approved can be classified as approvable and non-approvable. Approvable means that the respirators potentially meet the design criteria as set out in Part II. Non-Approvable respirators do not have a chance of being approved because they do not meet the basic specifications.

In addition to OSHA requirements for testing and approval, there is also the joint NIOSH/OSHA standard completion program which forms the basis for Respirator Decision Logic [3]. The purpose of decision logic is to provide the necessary criteria to support the selection of proper respiratory protection. It is a step-by-step procedure which eliminates inappropriate respirators and eventually leads to the correct choice of equipment. Protection factors are the criteria used to determine to what maximum concentrations the selected respirator may be worn. Reference to this NIOSH/OSHA Respiratory Decision Logic and the 30 CFRII should be made when respiratory protection equipment is being selected for the first time.

Thus, there are specific OSHA requirements for respirator approvals, including fit testings, respirator usage, care and maintenance, training and fitting, program administration, and surveillance and program evaluation.

From time to time, OSHA has changed its requirements for qualitative and quantitative fit testings of respirators used for the protection against a specific toxic substance. For example:

On November 12, 1982, OSHA amended its lead standard to permit the use of three qualitative fit testing (QLFT) procedures for respirators used to protect employees exposed to lead. The three protocols use either isoamyl acetate, saccharin, or irritant smoke (stannic oxychloride) and may be used only for airborne lead concentrations of up to 50 $\mu g/m^3$.

OSHA's lead standard, issued in 1978, originally required that only quantitative fit-testing (QNFT) be used to assess respirator protection effectiveness.

OSHA estimated that the QNFT requirement would have cost employers up to $6.8 million per year, but that the amended rule which gives employers the choice of QNFT and QLFT would cost $500,000 annually.

Similarly, NIOSH constantly issues a number of notices and warnings concerning respirators. For example:

On February 11, 1983 NIOSH advised the discontinuance of the Robertshaw RAM-5 combination 5-minute emergency escape self-contained breathing apparatus and supplied-air respirator (MSHA/NIOSH Approval Number TC-13F-64). This was due to problems which shortened service-time of the self-contained air supply.

On March 23, 1983 NIOSH advised that the Robertshaw RAM-5 (MSHA/NIOSH Approval Number TC-13F-64) could now be used if the testing and inspection procedure, as recommended by the manufacturer, showed no defects were present. In the event a RAM-5 respirator does not perform satisfactorily during recommended tests, it should then be returned to the distributor.

On March 3, 1983 NIOSH followed up an announcement of November 15, 1982 concerning the protection factors of certain powered air-purifying respirators (PAPRs). The current notice states that for both the 3M (Approval Number TC-21C-246) and Racal (Approval Number TC-21C-212), approximately 133 of the observed workplace-protection factors were below 1000. Approximately 95% of the observed workplace protection factors for both the 3M and Racal PAPRs exceeded 33.

On March 15, 1983 NIOSH advised that users of Robertshaw model 3000 compressed-air escape self-contained breathing apparatus (NIOSH Approval Number TC-13F-28) should inspect those respirators monthly in accordance with the manufacturers' instructions. This is in response to two reports of problems due to the gradual leakage of air from these respirators.

## A SUMMARY OF BRITISH STANDARDS INSTITUTION REQUIREMENTS

British Standards, like other respiratory standards, are designed to assist in the selection of respirators for protection against atmospheric contaminants, such as dust and gas, and against oxygen deficiency.

British Standards have been revised several times under the following designations:

BS 2091   Respirators for protection against harmful dusts, gases, and scheduled agricultural chemicals [4]
BS 4555   High-efficiency dust respirators [5]
BS 4558   Positive-pressure powered dust respirators [6]
BS 4667   Breath apparatus [7]
          Part 1.   Closed-circuit breathing apparatus
          Part 2.   Open-circuit breathing apparatus
          Part 3.   Fresh-air hose and compressed air-line breathing apparatus

Part 4.   Escape breathing apparatus
BS 47711   Positive-pressure, powered dust hoods and blouses [8]

The Institution warns users of the standards to refer to the latest edition of these standards, including amendments.

In addition to the preceding standards, the Institution also published recommendations and specifications for fit test, selection, use, care and maintenance of respiratory protective equipment. For example, BS 6016 provides detailed specifications for filtering-facepiece dust respirators [9].

BS 4275 gives recommendations for the selective use and maintenance of respiratory protective equipment [10], and BS 4400 provides details for sodium chloride tests for respirator filters [11].

British Standards provide certification for a product created to ensure personal safety and quotes the following in their specification:

A license to use the Kitemark or Safety mark on or in relation to a product will be granted to any manufacturer or producer who demonstrates that he/ she can and will be able consistently to make that product to the requirements specified in the British Standard. His/her capability of doing so is initially assessed by inspection of his/her production process, quality control organization and test facilities, and by independent testing of a sample of the product against all the criteria of the relevant standard. The licensee is required to accept and to operate in accordance with a BSI scheme of supervision and control which identifies the minimum level of quality control to be exercised during manufacture and the tests to be carried out on the completed product. BSI carries out unannounced inspection visits to the manufacturer's works and audit-testing of the product, and may withdraw the license for any failure of the manufacturer to comply with the relevant standard or the requirements of the scheme of supervision and control. The presence of the mark on or in relation to a product is an assurance that the goods have been produced under a system of supervision, control and testing, operated during manufacture and including periodical inspection of the manufacturer's works, in accordance with the certification mark scheme of BSI.

Other countries just as Japan, Germany, Italy, etc., have standards for respiratory protection equipment which outline specification and performance requirements. In recent articles published in the October edition of the American Industrial Hygiene Association's Journal, C. Ryan, et al, have reviewed the basic requirements in international standards for respiratory protection equipment [12-14]. They concluded that current respirator standards could better meet the objectives of a respirator certification program if they were changed to better represent conditions of actual use and if properly selected test challenges were used to evaluate protection capacity.

It is essential that the worker familiarize himself with the regulatory requirements governing the use of respiratory protection equipment in his workplace. We recommend that you contact your local occupational health and safety agency for specific details on regulatory requirements for the use of respirators.

## CRITERIA FOR SELECTION

Under normal circumstances there are few manufacturing operations or maintenance procedures that require the use of a respirator. Ordinarily, it is more practical and less costly to use process-engineering controls, good work practices, and less toxic materials to maintain employee exposures at acceptable levels. All Occupational Health and Safety Acts in North America require that air-contamination levels be reduced to the lowest feasible level by engineering controls and process design. Where this is not possible, or while such controls are being implemented, the appropriate respirators may be used to protect employees.

Jobs that may require the use of respiratory-protection equipment include, but are not limited to, the following:

1. Grinding, cutting or otherwise machining of solid materials that may liberate significant quantities of uncontrolled dust.
2. Manufacturing operations that require entry into oxygen-deficient or potentially oxygen-deficient atmospheres.
3. Maintenance in areas processing, handling, storing, or disposing of potentially toxic materials.
4. Under emergency conditions (spills, leaks, etc.) for escape, rescue, repairs, or shutdown.

When respirators are used, it is essential that a respiratory protection program be established. Proper respirator selection can be one of the most difficult jobs for the health and safety professional in a respiratory-protection program. There are a number of different types of respiratory hazards and certain limitations to differentiate types of respirators. It is essential that the proper respirator be selected. Proper respirator selection is the choice of a device that fully protects the worker from the hazards to which he may be exposed, provides the greatest reliability possible, and will permit the worker to perform the job with the least amount of discomfort and fatigue.

Selection of the proper type of respirator for any given situation should require consideration of the following facts:

1. The nature of the hazard,
2. The characteristics of the hazardous operation or process,
3. The location of the hazardous area with respect to a safe area having respirable air,
4. The period of time for which respiratory protection may be required,

5. The activity of workers in the hazardous area,
6. The physical characteristics, functional capabilities, and limitations of respirators of various types,
7. The respirator fit factor and respirator fit.

## The Nature of the Hazard

The following conditions should be considered in the selection procedure.

1. Type of hazard
   a. Oxygen deficiency
   b. Contaminant
2. Physical properties (gas, vapor, dust, mist, fume)
3. Chemical properties
4. Physiological effects on the body
5. Actual concentration (average, peak) of the toxic material. Recognition and evaluation of the respiratory hazard is an essential part of selecting a respirator. Initial monitoring of the respiratory hazard must be carried out to obtain data needed for the selection of proper respiratory protection. This would include the identification of the type of respiratory hazard, the airborne concentration and the nature of the contaminant.
6. Established permissible time-weighted average or peak concentration of the toxic material.
7. Whether the concentration of toxic material presents a hazard which is immediately dangerous to life or health (IDLH). IDLH is defined as conditions that pose an immediate threat to life or health or an immediate threat of severe exposure to contaminants which are likely to have adverse cumulative or delayed effects on health. Two facts are considered when establishing IDLH concentrations.
   a. The worker must be able to escape without losing his life or suffering permanent health damage within 30 minutes.
   b. The worker must be able to escape without severe eye or respiratory irritation or other reactions that could inhibit escape.
   If the concentration is above the IDLH, only a highly reliable breathing apparatus, such as positive-pressure demand is allowed.
8. Warning Properties. Warning properties, such as odor, eye irritation, and respiratory irritation that rely for detection upon human senses, are not foolproof. However, they do provide some indication to the wearer that the service-life of the cartridge or canister is reaching the end, the facepiece is not fitted properly, or there is some other respirator malfunction. Warning properties may be assumed to be adequate when the effects of odor, taste, or irritation from the substance can be detected and are persistent at concentrations or at below the

permissible exposure level. If the odor or irritating threshold of the material is many times greater than the permissable-exposure limit, the substance is considered to have poor warning properties, and air-supplied respirators must be specified. Table 2.3, Chapter 2, contains pertinent information on odor-threshold limit values for a number of contaminants.

9.  Skin absorption of the contaminant must be considered. Skin protection must be provided when information is available indicating possible systematic injury or death resulting from absorbance of a gas or vapor through the skin. This may take the form of impervious coverings or supplied-air suits.

10. Eye irritation must also be looked at. Eye protection may be required in the case of certain concentrations of acid gases and organic vapors. Full-face respirators may be needed to aid in the protection of the eyes as well as the respiratory tract.

## The Characteristics of the Hazardous Operations or Process

In selecting the proper respirator the operation or process in which the respirator has to be worn must be closely scrutinized. Workers' activities, the characteristics of the operation or process, and work area characteristics must be considered in the selection procedure. Materials used, including raw materials, end products and by-products must be known in order to select the proper respirator. Any modification in the operation should be investigated because this may change the hazard and/or the degree of the hazard and thus a different respirator may be needed.

## The Location of the Hazardous Area

Are there safe areas where respirable air is present near the hazardous area? This should be considered when selecting the proper respiratory equipment. Depending on the location of the hazardous area, the need to escape in case of a leak or accident, and the possibility of the need for rescue may influence the type of respirator that is needed.

## Respirator Usage Time

Consideration must be given to the application of the respirator. Is it routine, non-routine, emergency, escape or rescue use? The length of time the respirator has to be worn will influence selection. Lightweight, comfortable respirators should be selected for routine wearing over long periods of time during the work shift.

## Worker Activity in the Hazardous Area

Worker activity and location in the hazardous operation should be examined. The selection of a proper respirator will be influenced by whether the work rate is light, medium or heavy and whether the worker is in the area continuously or irregularly.

## Respirator Characteristics, Capabilities, and Limitations

The characteristics, capabilities, and limitations of different types of respirators (detailed in Chapter 2) must be considered in the selection procedure.

The preceding six conditions must be considered when selecting the proper respiratory equipment to ensure the protection of the workers in the hazardous work area. Figure 3.1 summarizes the steps necessary in selecting the proper respirator. Specific respirator selection sequences are summarized in Tables 3.1, 3.2, and 3.3 [15].

## FITTING

Considering the characteristics of the hazard involved, and the capabilities and limitations of the respirator will allow for the selection of a proper type of respirator, but it will not ensure that the worker is protected. Proper face-fit of the respirator is the last factor to consider in the selection procedure and it is essential. The wearing of a poorly fitting respirator may be more dangerous than not wearing a respirator at all. The worker may think he is protected when in reality he is not. The following factors affect the fit of a respirator:

1. Design of the respirator,
2. Facial features and facial hair,
3. Change in physical features, and
4. Training.

The term *Protection Factor* has been used for many years to refer to the measure of respirator performance. This term has been misused throughout the past few years. The Protection Factor for a respirator is a fraction calculated as the amount of contaminant outside the respirator as compared to that inside the respirator. This factor is the number assigned to a particular type of respirator or to an entire class of respirator, representing the degree of protection that the respirator is thought to provide for the majority of users. Protection Factor determinations are not made for an individual respirator wearer. Much research has been done to assign pro-

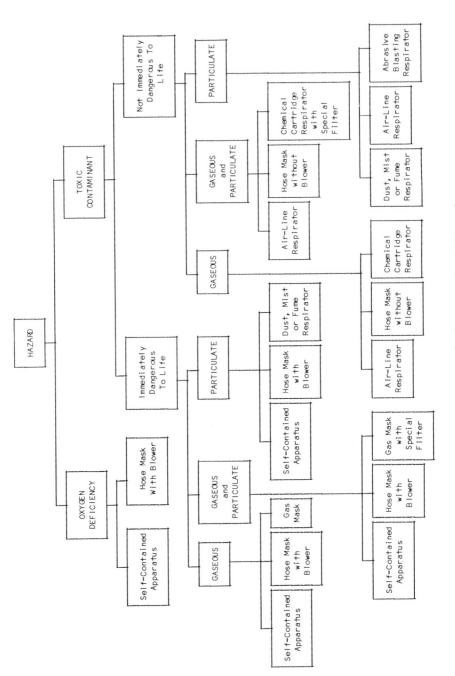

**Figure 3.1** Respirator selection according to hazard.

Table 3.1   For respiratory protection against gases or vapors

| Application | Selection Sequence |
|---|---|
| Routine Use | (a) Consider absorption through the skin;<br><br>(b) If the contaminant has poor warning properties, eliminate all air-purifying respirators;<br><br>(c) If eye irritation occurs, eliminate or restrict the use of a half-mask respirator;<br><br>(d) If concentration is greater than IDLH or LEL, eliminate all but positive-pressure SCBA and combination positive-pressure SCBA;<br><br>(e) List suitable respirators by condition of use and type. |
| Entry and escape from unknown concentrations | Use positive-pressure SCBA or combination positive-pressure supplied-air respirator with positive-pressure SCBA |
| Firefighting | Use positive-pressure SCBA. |
| Escape | Use gas mask or escape-SCBA. |

tection factors to the various types of respirators. Table 3.4 illustrates the Protection Factors assigned by the Las Alamos study and these have been generally accepted [16].

Two other terms which are used to describe the respirator's protection ability are *Fit Factor* and *Field Performance Factor*.

*Fit Factor* is the measure of the sealing of a respirator to the face of the wearer, as determined by the quantitative fit-test. It is the ratio of the concentration of the test atmosphere outside the respirator to the concentration inside. Fit Factor is only a measure of the effectiveness of the seal between the face and the respirator. This factor is assigned to a particular individual and respirator facepiece based on the individual testing. It gives some indication of the expected performance of the respirator on the wearer in the workplace.

The *Field Performance Factor* is a measure of the actual protection provided by the respirator while it is worn in the workplace. The Field Performance Factor is the ratio of the contaminant outside the respirator to

Table 3.2    For respiratory penetration against particulates

| Application | Selection Sequence |
|---|---|
| Routine Use | (a) Consider absorption through the skin;<br><br>(b) If eye irritation occurs, eliminate or restrict use of the half-mask respirator;<br><br>(c) When the maximum permissable exposure is less than $0.5$ mg/m$^3$ eliminate dust, fume, and mist (DFM) respirators unless they are fitted with high-efficiency particulate air filters;<br><br>(d) If the concentration is greater than IDLH or LEL, eliminate all but positive-pressure SCBA and combination positive-pressure SCBA;<br><br>(e) List suitable respirators by condition of use and type. |
| Entry and escape from unknown concentrations | Use positive-pressure SCBA or combination positive-pressure supplied-air respirator with positive-pressure SCBA |
| Firefighting | Use positive-pressure SCBA. |

that on the inside. Factors that affect the Field Performance Factor include facepiece sealing, efficiency of the air-cleaning elements, training and attitude of the wearer, comfort of the respirator and ease of putting on and adjusting the respirator.

*Respirator Fit,* simply stated, is the ability of the device to interface with the wearer in such a manner as to prevent the workplace atmosphere from entering the wearer's respiratory system through that interface. When the contaminated atmosphere penetrates the interface and enters the wearer's breathing zone, exposure occurs. Assessment and control must be made of the exposure resulting from less than a perfect fit in order to effectively utilize respirators as a means to control airborne hazards. There is professional agreement on the need to assess and control respirator fit, but there is very little agreement on the methods to be used and control levels to be attained.

Currently there are four classes of methods to assess respirator fit:

Table 3.3   For respiratory penetration against a combination of gas or vapor and particulates

| Application | Selection Sequence |
|---|---|
| Routine Use | (a) Consider absorption through the skin; <br><br> (b) If the contaminant has poor warning properties or inadequate sorbent efficiency, eliminate all air-purifying respirators; <br><br> (c) Eliminate all respirators, except those with combination sorbent/ particulate filters; <br><br> (d) If eye irritation occurs, eliminate or restrict the use of the half-mask respirator; <br><br> (e) When the maximum permissible exposure is less than 0.05 mg/m$^3$, eliminate all respirators except those fitted with sorbent/high-efficiency particulate air filters; <br><br> (f) If the concentration is greater than IDLH or LEL, eliminate all but positive-pressure SCBA and combination positive-pressure SCBA; <br><br> (g) List suitable respirators by condition of use and type. |
| Entry and escape from unknown concentrations | Use positive-pressure SCBA or combination positive-pressure supplied-air respirator with positive-pressure SCBA |
| Firefighting | Use positive-pressure SCBA. |
| Escape | Gas mask or escape-SCBA. |

1. Positive-/Negative-Pressure Checks;
2. Qualitative Fit Tests;
3. Quantitative Fit Tests;
4. Protection-Factor Tests.

Recently, Semi-Quantitative Fit Tests have been introduced by OSHA as an alternative to Quantitative Fit Tests in the Lead Standard.

Table 3.4   Respirator protection factors

| Type Respirator | Facepiece[2] Pressure | Protec- tion Factor |
|---|---|---|
| I. Air-Purifying | | |
| A.Particulate[3] removing | | |
| Single-use[4], dust[5] | − | 5 |
| Quarter-mask, dust[6] | − | 5 |
| Half-mask, dust[6] | − | 10 |
| Half- or Quarter-mask, fume[7] | − | 10 |
| Half- or Quarter-mask, High-Efficiency[8] | − | 10 |
| Full Facepiece, High-Efficiency | − | 50 |
| Powered, High-Efficiency, all enclosures | + | 1,000 |
| Powered, dust or fume, all enclosures | + | $x$[9] |
| B.Gas and Vapour-Removing[10] | | |
| Half-Mask | − | 10 |
| Full Facepiece | − | 50 |
| | | |
| II. Atmosphere-Supplying | | |
| A.Supplied-Air | | |
| Demand, Half-mask | − | 10 |
| Demand, Full Facepiece | − | 50 |
| Hose Mask Without Blower, Full Facepiece | − | 50 |
| Pressure-Demand, Half-Mask[11] | + | 1,000 |
| Pressure-Demand, Full Facepiece[12] | + | 2,000 |
| Hose Mask With Blower, Full Facepiece | − | 50 |
| Continuous Flow, Half-Mask[11] | + | 1,000 |
| Continuous Flow, Full Facepiece[12] | + | 2,000 |
| Continuous Flow, Hood, Helmet, or Suit[13] | + | 2,000 |
| B.Self-Contained Breathing Apparatus (SCBA) | | |
| Open-Circuit, Demand, Full Facepiece | − | 50 |
| Open-Circuit, Pressure-demand, Full Facepiece | + | 10,000[14] |
| Closed-Circuit, Oxygen Tank-type, | | |
| Full Facepiece | − | 50 |
| | | |
| III. Combination Respirator | | |
| A.Any combination of air-purifying and atmosphere-supplying respirator | Use minimum protection | |
| B.Any combination of supplied-air respirator and an SCBA | factor listed above for type of mode of operation | |

   Exception:  Combination supplied-air respirators, in
   pressure-demand or other positive pressure mode, with an
   auxiliary self-contained air supply, and a full facepiece,
   should use the PF for pressure-demand SCBA.

1.  The overall protection afforded by a given respirator design (and
    mode of operation) may be defined in terms of its protection factor
    (PF).  The PF is a measure of the degree of protection afforded by a
    respirator, defined as the ratio of the concentration of contaminant
    in the ambient atmosphere to that inside the enclosure (usually
    inside the facepiece) under conditions of use.  Respirators should
    be selected so that the concentration inhaled by the wearer will not
    exceed the appropriate limit.  The recommended respirator PF's are
    selection and use guides, and should only be used when the employer
    has established a minimal acceptable respirator program as defined
    in Section 3 of the ANSI Z88.2-1969 Standard.

Table 3.4  *(continued)*

2. In addition to facepieces, this includes any type of enclosure or covering of the wearer's breathing zone, such as supplied-air hoods helmets, or suits.

3. Includes dusts, mists, and fumes only. Does not apply when gases or vapours are absorbed on particulates and may be volatized or for particulates volatile at room temperature. Example: Coke oven emissions.

4. Any single-use dust respirator (with or without valve) not specifically tested against a specified contaminant.

5. Singe-use dust respirators have been tested against asbestos and cotton dust and could be assigned a PF of 10 for these particulates.

6. Dust filter refers to a dust respirator approved by the silica dust test, and includes all types of media, that is, both nondegradable mechanical type media and degradable resin-impregnated wool felt or combination wool-synthetic felt media.

7. Fume filter refers to a fume respirator approved by the lead fume test. All types of media are included.

8. High-efficiency filter refers to a high-efficiency particulate respirator. The filter must be at least 99.97% efficient against 0.3 $\mu$m DOP to be approved.

9. To be assigned, based on dust or fume filter efficiency for specific contaminant.

10. For gases and vapors, a PF should only be assigned when published test data indicate the cartridge or canister has adequate sorbent efficiency and service life for a specific gas or vapour. In addition, the PF should not be applied in gas or vapour concentrations that are: 1) immediately dangerous to life, 2) above the lower explosive limit, and 3) cause eye irritation when using a half-mask.

11. A positive pressure supplied-air respirator equipped with a half-mask facepiece may not be as stable on the face as a full facepiece. Therefore, the PF recommended is half that for a similar device equipped with a full facepiece.

12. A positive pressure supplied-air respirator equipped with a full facepiece provides eye protection but is not approved for use in atmospheres immediately dangerous to life. It is recognized that the facepiece leakage, when a positive pressure is maintained, should be the same as an SCBA operated in the positive pressure mode. However, to emphasize that it basically is not for emergency use, the PF is limited to 2,000.

13. The design of the supplied-air hood, suit, or helmet (with a minimum of 6 cfm of air) may determine its overall efficiency and protection. For example, when working with the arms over the head, some hoods draw the contaminant into the hood breathing zone. This may be overcome by wearing a short hood under a coat or overalls. Other limitations specified by the approval agency must be considered before using in certain types of atmospheres.

Table 3.4    *(continued)*

14. The SCBA operated in the positive pressure mode has been tested on a
    selected 31-man panel and the facepiece leakage recorded as less
    than 0.01% penetration. Therefore, a PF of 10,000+ is recommended.
    At this time, the lower limit of detection 0.01% does not warrant
    listing a higher number. A positive pressure SCBA for an unknown
    concentration is recommended. This is consistent with the 10,000+
    that is listed. It is essential to have an emergency device for use
    in unknown concentrations. A combination supplied-air respirator in
    pressure-demand or other positive pressure mode, with auxiliary
    self-contained air supply is also recommended for use in unknown
    concentrations of contaminants immediately dangerous to life. Other
    limitations, such as skin absorption of HCN or titrium, must be
    considered.

## Positive-/Negative-Pressure Checks

Pressure checks are the most frequently used methods. They are the least precise and are applicable only to tight-fitting respiratory inlet coverings. The positive-pressure method involves having the wearer close the outlet of the respirator (Figure 3.2). The wearer checks either for outward leakage around the sealing edge or the length of time the pressure is maintained in order to judge the adequacy of the seal.

The negative-pressure method involves the wearer closing the inlet of the respirator and then inhaling, creating a relatively high negative pressure inside the facepiece (Figure 3.3). The same criteria as those of the positive-pressure check are used by the wearer to judge the adequacy of the seal.

Although these checks only detect large leaks, they are the only methods that are easily administered by the user himself and thus are the most feasible methods for checking fit each time the respirator is put on.

**Figure 3.2** Positive-pressure face-fit test on a dual-cartridge respirator.

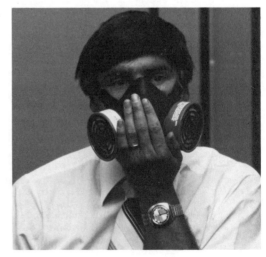

**Figure 3.3** Negative-pressure face-fit test on a disposable respirator.

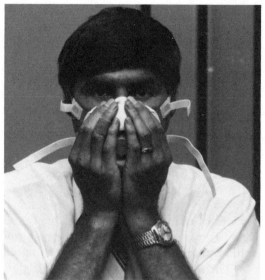

The advantages of these tests are that they are simple and quick, can be carried out by the wearer himself and can be performed after each donning of the respirator during a workshift.

The limitation of these tests is that only large leaks can be detected. Care must be taken not to force the respirator against the face of the wearer, thereby creating an unrealistic sealing force with the result of low leakage.

## Qualitative Fit Tests

Qualitative fit tests are frequently used in industry. They provide a valid assessment of fit for negative-pressure respirators used for protection against toxic contaminants.

There are three qualitative methods, and all generate a test atmosphere around the respirator attempting to concentrate it around the sealing area. If a significant leak exists, the wearer senses the presence of the test agent; if the test agent is not detected the respirator is judged to have an adequate fit.

### Irritant Smoke Test

This method is commonly used with air-supplied respirators or air-purifying respirators equipped with high efficiency air-purifying elements. The 'smoke' is generated by aspiring moist room air through a stannic chloride ventilation test tube. The smoke consists of HCl on a very small oxide particle and it is directed around the sealing surface of the respirator. If a leak is present, the wearer detects it by reacting to the irritation, usually with an involuntary cough.

The main advantage of this method is that it usually evokes an involuntary response in the form of a cough or a sneeze. The likelihood of this giving a false indication of proper fit is reduced. The main limitation with irritant smoke is that the test must be performed with caution because the aerosol is highly irritating to the eyes, skin and mucous membrane.

### Isoamyl Acetate or Banana Oil Method

Isoamyl acetate is a liquid having a strong smell of bananas. The test atmosphere is usually generated by slowly passing a swab wet with the chemical around the sealing surface of the respirator (Figure 3.4). The test atmosphere challenges each general sealing area of the respirator during the inhalation cycle of respiration—the time when leakage is most likely to occur. To prepare for this test, the respirator must be supplied or equipped with a purifying element capable of removing organic vapors.

The major limitation of this method is that it depends on human senses (smell) and odor thresholds vary widely among individuals.

### Saccharin Test

This method, developed by 3M, may be used on any air-supplied or air-purifying respirator equipped with any air-purifying element approved to remove particulate hazard.

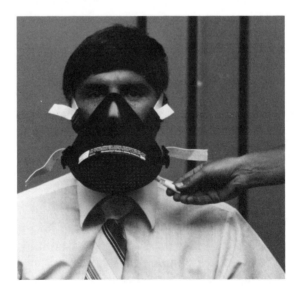

**Figure 3.4**    Isoamyl acetate qualitative face fit test.

The test is generated by nebulizing a saccharin/water solution (Figure 3.5). The water evaporates leaving a small particle, approximately 2.0 microns in diameter. Again, the sealing edge of the respirator is challenged as before, and the wearer breathes through his mouth throughout the test. If a significant leak is present, the wearer will detect a sweet taste.

As with the isoamyl-acetate method the major limitation of this method is that it depends on an individual's ability to taste saccharin.

## Semi-Quantitative Fit Tests

Semi-quantitative fit tests were designed to offer an alternative to the difficult and costly quantitative fit test methods as they applied to the OSHA Lead Standard. Two methods have been proposed: one designed by DuPont uses Isoamyl Acetate, and the other, by 3M, uses Saccharin.

In principle, both methods are the same. Each one involves, first of all, pre-screening to determine whether the subject is sensitive to a low, known concentration of the test chemical. If he is sensitive to the concentration, then a qualitative fit test is carried out. If he is not, then they will not be tested using this method. Therefore, false fits are eliminated.

OSHA recently published a revision to the fit testing requirements of the Lead Standard (29CFR 1910.1025(f)[3]). In addition to quantitative fit testing, OSHA will now permit three methods of qualitative fit testing for

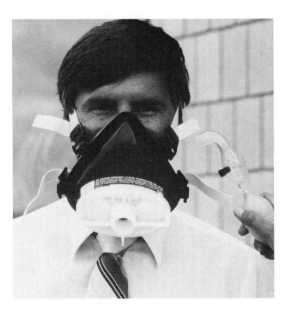

**Figure 3.5** Saccharin qualitative face-fit test.

assigning respirators to lead-exposed employees. The isoamyl-acetate method, the saccharin-solution-aerosol method, or the irritant-smoke method can be used for testing half-mask respirators only. To comply with the Lead Standard, protocol must be followed exactly.

### Quantitative Fit Tests

Theoretically these tests should provide an accurate, objective measurement of fit for all types of respirators. The quantitative fit test is intended to yield a numerical measurement of actual leakage.

Quantitative tests were developed in the early sixties as a laboratory technique for evaluating respirator fit. Until recently, the equipment and technique were so complex that they remained laboratory tools only. Portable equipment is now available, and this has opened the technique to the industrial user.

There are two principal methods currently being used in North America: sodium chloride and dioctylphthalate (DOP). Other tests use methylene blue, paraffin oil, silica, ethylene gas, or Freon.

DOP, the most common, is used in the form of a polydispersed aerosol as a test agent and is detected with a light scattering photometer. Sodium chloride is also used in the form of a polydispersed aerosol and is detected with a flame photometer.

In order to carry out the quantitative fit tests, the atmosphere is continuously measured inside the respirator through a probe in the respirator facepiece, and at the same time it is measured outside the respirator (Figure 3.6). The wearer is required to stand in a chamber where the test material

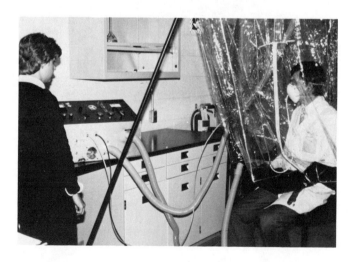

**Figure 3.6**   Quantitative face-fit test: portable booth.

atmosphere is generated. The leakage is expressed as a percentage of the test atmosphere outside the respirator. The advantages of quantitative fit testing are as follows:

1. It is an excellent training tool to teach the wearer to don, position, and adjust the facepiece for reliable, repeatable, and adequate protection through the instantaneous response of the detector to penetrations of ambient air into the mask.
2. It provides instantaneous feedback of changes in facefit-sealing efficiency caused by movements and adjustments to the facepiece.
3. It gives the wearer increased confidence in the assigned respirator.
4. It provides documented results to the respirator-selection process.
5. It provides a means to assess variations in fit on the individual, and over periods of time.
6. It reduces the subjectivity in the selection process by generating data for each respirator-wearer and allowing the user to compare results.

The disadvantages of quantitative fit tests are as follows:

1. They are very costly. Commercially available portable units range in price from $11,000 to $18,000.
2. They are a very time-consuming operation.
3. A skilled operator is required to effectively operate and maintain the equipment. It may take many months of operator training and experience before useful data can be obtained.
4. Since the concentration of the test agent inside the respirator varies sinusoidally with the frequency of the breathing rate, and since leakage is usually quantified by peak height, large variations in response time can lead to large variations in measured leakage values.
5. Due to the complex nature of quantitative fit tests techniques, some people may downplay other aspects of the complete respirator program. Some users may feel that as long as they have data to show that the respirator fits adequately they may neglect care and maintenance, or subject the respirator to rigorous wear.
6. The respirator which is tested is not the one worn by workers in the field. It is assumed that different respirators of the same model will be similar. This may not always be true, due to quality control deficiencies during manufacturing.
7. As the name implies, the test determines fit only. It may be dangerous to use quantitative fit tests to derive protection factors.

Once the proper respirator has been selected to match the job hazards and conditions, there are three essential elements which contribute to how well the respirator will protect the user:

1.  The condition of the equipment;
2.  How well the respirator fits the wearer; and
3.  How long the respirator is worn in the contaminated area.

The condition of the equipment depends on the quality of the cleaning and maintenance program. If the respirator is not properly maintained contaminated air can leak into the mask.

The fit of the respirator on the wearer's face, as we have discussed in this chapter, can be expressed as *Fit Factor* and the face seal's protection level can be assessed either by qualitative or quantitative methods.

The third consideration involves the worker's willingness to wear the respirator and the time he wears it in the contaminated area. This is considered the *Wear Factor* which is a measure of the percent of time the mask is actually being worn during the work shift [17]. Even though a respirator has a high Fit Factor and does an effective job of filtering out the contaminant while being worn, overall protection is drastically reduced by neglecting to wear the respirator in the contaminated area even for brief periods of time. Figure 3.7 shows how dramatically this protection drops off as the "non-worn" time increases [17].

The relationship of the Fit Factor and the Wear Factor to the Protection Factor can best be illustrated by examples.

In an 8-hour exposure at 10x PEL, a respirator with Fit Factor = 1.000 that is worn 95% of the shift (not worn for 24 minutes) will have a Protection Factor equaling 20. If the respirator is worn 98% of the shift (not worn for 10 minutes), the Protection Factor is 50. On the other hand, a respirator with a Fit Factor of 100 that is worn 99% of the shift (not worn 5 minutes) will also have a Protection Factor of 50. Table 3.5 summarizes the Wear Factor results for different fit factors and percent of time worn. These examples show that keeping a respirator on significantly affects how much protection is being provided.

The reasons why workers remove their respirators are numerous and include: the respirators are heavy and/or uncomfortable; they are difficult to breathe through, difficult to speak through, or too hot. Any selection of a proper respirator must consider these objections in order to ensure a high percentage of respirator-wear time.

In summary then, there are many factors which must be carefully considered in respirator selection. The nature and extent of the hazard should be determined. The operation and work activities must be studied. The respirator's limitations and characteristics must be weighed with care, taking into account whether IDLH conditions exist and/or whether or not the contaminant has poor warning properties. Finally, you must make sure that the respirator provides the required and proper face seal and degree of protection. All these factors and possibilities must be carefully examined by the health and safety professional when selecting any respiratory protection de-

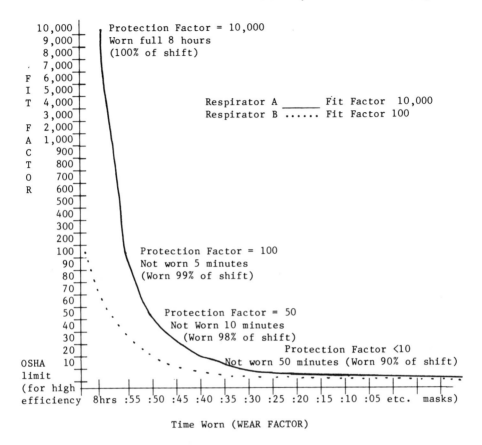

**Figure 3.7**  Wear factor vs. fit factor.

vice. Even when all of these factors are considered, the worker must wear the respirator because, as we have seen, when the respirator is removed for a short period of time protection is reduced significantly.

## REFERENCES

1.  Federal Register, Vol. 37, Number 202, Tables 29 and 30.
2.  *NIOSH Certified Equipment List,* OHHS (NIOSH) Publication No. 80-144, Cincinnati (1980).
3.  Pritchard, J.A., "A Guide to Industrial Respiratory Protection," DHEW (NIOSH) Publication No. 76-189, Appendix F.
4.  British Standards Institution. *Specification for Respirator for Protection Against Harmful Dusts, Gases, and Schedule Agricultural Chemicals.* British Standards House BS 2091, London, England (1978).

Table 3.5   Wear factor

| FIT FACTOR | 80 | 90 | 95 | 100 |
|---|---|---|---|---|
| 10 | 2.80 | 1.90 | 1.45 | 1.00 |
| 25 | 2.32 | 1.36 | 0.88 | 0.40 |
| 50 | 2.16 | 1.18 | 0.69 | 0.20 |
| 100 | 2.08 | 1.09 | 0.595 | 0.10 |
| 1000 | 2.008 | 1.009 | 0.509 | 0.01 |
| INF | 2.00 | 1.00 | 0.50 | 0.00 |

5.  British Standards Institution. *Specification for High Efficiency Dust Respirators*. British Standards House BS 4555, London, England (1970).
6.  British Standards Institution. *Specification for Positive Pressure Powered Dust Respirator*. British Standards House BS 4558, London, England (1972).
7.  British Standards Institution. *Specification for Breathing Apparatus*. British Standards House BS 4667, London, England (1974).
8.  British Standards Institution. *Specification for Positive Pressure Powered Dust Hoods and Blouses*. British Standards House BS 47711, London, England (1974).
9.  British Standards Institution. *Specification for Filtering Facepiece Dust Respirator*. British Standards House BS 6016, London, England (1974).
10. British Standards Institution. *Recommendations for the Selection, Use and Maintenance of Respiratory Protectory Equipment*. British Standards House BS 4275, London, England (1974).
11. British Standards Institution. *Method for Sodium Chloride Particulate Test for Respiratory Filters*. British Standards House BS 4400, London, England (1972).
12. Ryan, C., Breysse, P.N., White, N., and Corn, M.: "Critical Review of International Standards for Respiratory Protective Equipment—I. Respiratory Protective Equipment for Particulate-Laden Atmospheres," *American Industrial Hygiene Association Journal* 44:756–761 (1983).
13. Breysse, P.N., White, N., Ryan, C.M., and Corn, M.: "Critical Review of International Standards for Respiratory Protective Equipment—II. Gas and Vapor Removal Efficiency and Fit Testing," *American Industrial Hygiene Association Journal* 44:762–767 (1983).
14. Breysse, P.N., White, N., Ryan, C.M., and Corn, M.: "Critical Review of International Standards for Respiratory Protective Equipment—III. Practical Performance Tests," *American Industrial Hygiene Association Journal* 44:768–773 (1983).

15. Canadian Standards Association. Standard Z94.4-M1982, *Selection, Care and Use of Respirators*, Appendix H. Canadian Standards Association, Rexdale, Canada (1982).
16. Pritchard, J.A., "A Guide to Industrial Respiratory Protection," DHEW (NIOSH) Publication No. 76-189, Pg. 54–56 (1979).
17. 3M Bulletin. *Job Health Highlight*, Vol. 1, #3, August (1983).

# 4

# *Administration and Training*

Chapters 2 and 3 have discussed different types of respirators available for use and the selection criteria used to choose the proper respirator. In order to assure that workers' health is being protected, a respiratory protection program must be established. This will be discussed in more detail in Chapter 7. This chapter will discuss two important components of the total program: Administration and Training.

In order for the respiratory program to be effective, the administration of the total system and the training of all people covered by the program must play a major role. Someone must be put in charge of the implementation and continuous administration of the respirator program. Respirators are misused and will continue to be misused unless an effective training component is incorporated into the program.

## ADMINISTRATION

In order that a respirator program be properly established—be started on the right foot—and be effective on an ongoing basis, written standard operating procedures must be established. These procedures should contain all the necessary information needed to maintain an effective respirator program and should be tailored to the user's requirements. The format of written procedures will vary, and should vary, since the requirements in different facilities vary. The written standard operating procedures should address the following topics:

1. Guidance for selection of the appropriate respirator.
2. Detailed procedures for:
   a. Cleaning, disinfecting, and storing;
   b. Inspecting, repairing, and replacing;
   c. Fit testing by the wearer and the tester;
   d. Purchasing of the proper respirator;
   e. Issuing of correct respirators;
   f. Training of the wearer, supervisor, and other appropriate personnel.

3.  Instructions for respirator use in emergencies.
4.  Guidelines for medical surveillance of workers.
5.  Procedures for evaluating the respirator program's effectiveness.

In order to ensure a proper respiratory protection program and that the procedures are written and adhered to, the responsibility for the entire program must be assigned to one person, a program administrator. The exact person to whom this will be assigned will vary from one organization to another. In a large organization there may be a number of personnel (such as Safety and Security, Maintenance, Industrial Relations, Industrial Hygiene, etc.) involved in the program, but all should report to one administrator. In a small shop, the administrator may be the only person involved in the entire program.

The program administrator must have sufficient knowledge, gained by training and experience, to develop and implement the respiratory protection program. He may have a background in safety, industrial hygiene, health care or engineering.

The major role of the administrator is to supervise and coordinate. He is responsible for written procedures and their revision when changes take place in the type of hazard present, the process, etc. The administrator must be knowledgeable in the state of the art respiratory protection and must change the program if needs change. Essentially, the administrator should:

1.  Establish a respirator program that meets the needs of the employer and employees;
2.  Ensure that it is carried out satisfactorily;
3.  Ensure that it remains effective by continued examination and modification where needed.

Once the respirator program has been established, it is essential that it be evaluated periodically (at a minimum, annually), to ensure adequate protection of the worker. This evaluation should be carried out by the administrator or someone outside of the program who is knowledgeable in the area of respiratory protection. Written procedures should be reviewed during the evaluation and changed where necessary. Operation of the program should be reviewed to ensure that proper types of respirators are issued and used; the respirators are properly worn and maintained; the respirators are inspected; and the respirators are properly stored.

During the evaluation the wearer should be consulted and wearer acceptance should be determined. Comfort, resistance to breathing, fatigue, interference with vision, interference with communications, restrictions of movement, interference with job performance, and confidence in respirator effectiveness are things that should be discussed with the wearer.

Biological and medical monitoring, where applicable, may be used to evaluate the effectiveness of the respirator and, where such data is available, should be reviewed during the evaluation process.

The results of the program evaluation should be presented in a written report and, if modifications are necessary, the plan of action to be implemented must also be included in the report.

In summary, in order to ensure the proper set-up, implementation and continuation of an effective respiratory protection program, an administrator must be appointed and he must be responsible for the entire program. Also, the support of upper management must be given to ensure a long-lived program.

## TRAINING

Selecting the proper respirator is one of the most important steps in ensuring the protection of the workers in a contaminated environment. Giving the respirator to the worker without teaching him how to use it reduces the probability of proper protection. A training program must be an integral part of any respiratory protection program. This applies to any size facility, whether only several people wear respirators occasionally, or a thousand workers wear them daily. One should not expect the wearer to know what to do with a respirator, even the simplest model, unless he is trained.

It has been shown that if a respirator is not worn in the contaminated area for even a short period of time the total protection offered by the respirator is drastically reduced. The role of a training program is to educate the wearer as to why the respirator is needed and how to wear it properly. If the employee wears the respirator all the time he needs to, the necessary protection is provided.

Table 4.1 shows the probability of respirators being worn given the approach of the employer to the implementation of the program. The education of the employees is vital to a successful program and this factor cannot be downplayed.

Table 4.1  Respirator use success

| Method of Implementation | Resulting Success Prediction | Meaning |
|---|---|---|
| By Decree | Doubtful | Open to question – imputes failure |
| By Persuasion | Dubious | Hesitation – Mistrust |
| By Incentive | Perhaps | Possibly but not Certainly and Maybe |
| By Education | Probably | Supported by evidence strong enough to establish presumption but not proof |
| By all of the above | Likely | Having a high probability of occurring. |

Who should be trained? The following people should be put through the respiratory protection training program:

1.   The wearer,
2.   The supervisor of the wearer,
3.   The person issuing respirators,
4.   The person performing the fit testing, and
5.   The person maintaining and repairing the respirators.

Not all of these people need to be trained in all aspects of respiratory protection, but certainly the wearer and his supervisor should be exposed to the entire program.

The wearer should receive the most thorough training. This training should convey a very clear picture to the wearer, as to why he should wear a respirator. At the end of the training session the wearer should be convinced that he needs to wear and maintain the respirator to protect his health. The wearer training should cover the following at a minimum:

1.   The nature, extent, and effect of respiratory hazards to which the person is being exposed.
2.   An explanation as to the reasons why respirators need to be used in place of other control methods.
3.   The operation, limitations, and capabilities of the selected respirator(s) must be covered.
4.   Instructions in procedures for inspecting, donning, wearing and removing, checking the fit and seal of respirators have to be explained.
5.   Each wearer must be given an opportunity in the training session to handle the respirator(s), to try on, check the fit, and remove them.
6.   Proper maintenance and storage procedures must be covered.
7.   Instructions in how to deal with emergency situations must be included.

The wearer's supervisor also needs to be trained. His training is basically the same as that of the wearer with the inclusion of the following additional points:

1.   The structure and operation of the entire respiratory protection program,
2.   The legal requirements pertinent to the use of respirators,
3.   The monitoring of respirator use, and
4.   The issuance of respirators.

The person(s) assigned to the task of issuing respirators should be given adequate training and written instructions to ensure that the correct respirator is issued for each application, in accordance with written standard operating procedures.

The person or persons responsible for performing fit tests should be trained in the proper procedure for carrying ıt the testing. He should be knowledgeable of the different brands and types of respirators used in his workplace and their specific applications.

Adequate training should be given to the personnel who are assigned the responsibility of maintaining and repairing the respirators.

It is essential to retrain all personnel involved in the respirator program. Each person should be annually retrained in the appropriate procedures that he needs to ensure that proper effective protection is being provided.

The administrator must set up a record-keeping system for the training program. This system should include the following records as a minimum:

1.   Who has been trained;
2.   When they received the training;
3.   What training sections they received;
4.   What results were obtained from their fit testing (is there any type of respirator which they cannot wear and why);
5.   Results of any medical testing (may indicate types of respirator they cannot wear due to health reasons. Also will indicate if respirator they are wearing is providing the necessary protection);
6.   Where the person works;
7.   What hazards the person is exposed to;
8.   What type(s) of respirator the person wears;
9.   How long the person wears the respirator during the workshift.

In order for a respiratory protection program to be successful, employee acceptance of the wearing of respiratory devices is vital. This acceptance deals more with human relations, and the education and training become key factors in motivating employees to use respirators correctly.

# 5

# *Maintenance and Care*

An integral part of a good respiratory protection program is the proper maintenance and care of the respirator. The purpose of a respirator is to prevent the inhalation of contaminant air. A serious problem may exist if a wearer dons a poorly maintained or malfunctioning respirator. He feels protected because the respirator is being worn, when in fact the contaminant is being inhaled and serious consequences may result. Each respirator, regardless of the type, must be properly maintained at the level of its original effectiveness. An acceptable program of maintenance and care must include:

1. Cleaning and sanitizing,
2. Inspection, testing and repair,
3. Storage, and
4. Record keeping.

It is an absolute must that any defective or non-functioning respirator be removed from use until repaired. If the respirator cannot be repaired then it must be discarded.

## CLEANING AND SANITIZING

Cleaning and sanitizing procedures must be included in the respirator protection program and must be part of the wearer's training program. Routinely used respirators should be cleaned and disinfected daily. On the other hand, emergency-use respirators and occasionally used respirators should be cleaned after each use.

In facilities where wearers are assigned individual respirators and are responsible for their own cleaning and disinfecting, each wearer must be thoroughly trained in cleaning and sanitizing procedures. In large establishments where a large number of respirators are used routinely, it may be practical to establish a centralized respirator-cleaning area manned by specially trained personnel.

A suggested procedure for cleaning and sanitizing is as follows:

113

1. All removable components (filters, cartridges, diaphragms, valves, etc.) are removed and inspected. Any defective part is repaired or discarded.
2. Wash the components in a 50°C water with a mild detergent or with a cleaner recommended by the manufacturer. A stiff bristle brush can be used to aid in the removal of any dirt. Care must be taken not to damage any of the components.
3. Rinse the components thoroughly in clean, warm (50°C) running water and drain.
4. Immerse the respirator components for 2 minutes in one of the following sanitizing solutions:
   a. Hypochlorite solution (50 ppm. of chlorine) made by adding approximately 1 ml. of laundry bleach to 1 liter of water at 50°C; or
   b. Aqueous solution of iodine (50 ppm. of iodine) made by adding approximately 0.8 ml. of tincture of iodine to 1 liter of water at 50°C.
5. Rinse all components thoroughly in clean warm (50°C) running water and drain.
6. Dry components with a clean lint-free cloth or air-dry.
7. Reassemble facepieces, replacing filters, cartridges or canisters where necessary.
8. Test the respirator to ensure that all components work properly.

In the case of disposable respirators which are reusable, the cleaning and sanitizing procedure is somewhat different and easier because there is no disassembling and reassembling involved. If the disposable respirator is to be kept for reuse then the face seal area must be wiped with water and a mild detergent or an alcohol wipe. It is then dried and stored in a clean dry area. The disposable type of respirator can be considered essentially maintenance free.

## INSPECTION, TESTING, AND REPAIR

The wearer must routinely inspect his respirator before and after each use. This inspection should include checking the following:

1. Tightness of the connections;
2. Condition of component parts (facepiece, connecting tubes, filters, cylinders, head harness, valves, etc.);
3. End-of-service-life indicator;
4. Shelf-life dates;
5. Proper functioning of regulators, alarms, and other warning systems;
6. SCBA cylinders filled to specific working pressure;
7. Pliability and deterioration of rubber or other elastomeric parts.

Respirators used for emergency, rescue or non-routinely should be inspected at least monthly. All respirators should be inspected after being cleaned and sanitized. This will involve the inspection points as outlined above and the necessary testing to ensure that the respirator and its components are in proper working condition.

All damaged or faulty components must be repaired or replaced. When this is necessary the repair and replacement should be done by persons trained in proper respirator assembly. The proper parts should be used and the repair and replacement should be carried out as per the manufacturer's instructions. Substitution of parts from one brand or type of respirator to another invalidates NIOSH approval (or equivalent approvals) of the respirator.

## STORAGE

All respirators must be properly stored in order to protect them from the environment and the possibility of damage. This includes protection from dust, sunlight, extreme temperature (hot or cold), excessive moisture, and damaging chemicals. All types of respirators should be kept in a cabinet separate from the work environment in a clean-air area. There must be easy access to the storage cabinets for non-routine or emergency respirators in order to ensure the wearer is able to put on the necessary equipment to protect himself in the case of an emergency. These storage cabinets should be clearly marked. Routinely used respirators should not be stored in workbenches, tool boxes or lockers unless they are protected from contamination, distortion, and damage.

## RECORD KEEPING

Record keeping is essential to a good maintenance program for respirators. A record of all inspections performed on respirators should be maintained and should include:

1.  Date of use,
2.  Date of inspection,
3.  Physical condition of the respirator,
4.  Cleaning and sanitizing of respirator date,
5.  Repairs carried out,
6.  The tests performed and any corrective action taken.

These records should be maintained by the administrator of the respiratory protection program.

In summary then, proper maintenance and care of respirators and their components are very important in ensuring the protection of workers in the workplace. A good respiratory protection program must contain provisions for cleaning, disinfecting, inspecting and maintaining all respirators covered by the program. Failure to do so may jeopardize the health of workers.

# 6

# *Medical Supervision*

The three main purposes of medical supervision are: to fulfill legislative requirements; to determine fitness to work in the workplace; and to follow changes in the health status of employees over time and assess if a correlation exists between those changes and the working environment.

The use of a respirator, regardless of the type, imposes some physical discomfort and distress. The degree of distress is dependent on various factors such as:

1. *Breathing Resistance.* For example, air-purifying respirators make breathing more difficult. The special exhalation valve on an open-circuit pressure-demand respirator requires the wearer to exhale against significant resistance.
2. *Vision Limitation.* Vision is restricted to some extent with all devices and this can lead to tunnel vision or perceptual narrowing. This response can in turn lead to the production of anxiety in certain individuals above and beyond the stress induced by heavy physical work, e.g., firefighting.
3. *Movement Restriction.* Movement is restricted because of the cumbersome nature of some equipment. For example, if the wearer is using an airline respirator, he might have to drag up to 300 feet of hose around.
4. *Communication Restriction.* All respiratory equipment restricts communication. This can become unpleasant, and at times, add to existing stress.
5. *Weight.* All respiratory devices impose an extra burden on the wearer, but some heavier devices such as SCBA add even greater strain.
6. *Thermal Stress.* Covering the face with an impervious mask significantly impairs heat loss from the head. Depending upon the work activity, the sweat rate may increase by as much as 8 percent, but evaporation sweat loss may be reduced by 12 percent [1].
7. *Psychophysiological Effects.* A feeling of claustrophobia may develop in some wearers of respirators. Identifying those individuals who experience such problems is not always easy.

Now let us consider a worker suffering from emphysema who is required to wear air-purifying devices. It is not hard to visualize the severe complications he would develop. Similarly, diseases such as asthma and chronic bronchitis will severely limit respirator usage. Those who suffer from heart disease may find that any of the above-described factors accentuate their problems. Epileptic workers may rip off their masks while working in atmospheres immediately dangerous to life. It is therefore imperative to determine individual fitness or ability to wear respirators without aggravating a pre-existing medical problem. The following guidelines will assist in developing an effective medical surveillance program.

## THE EXAMINING PHYSICIAN

The examining physician has the responsibility for directing an effective health-surveillance medical program with major emphasis on prevention. In order to render a qualified opinion regarding respirator usage by an employee, the physician initially should obtain the following information:

- Type of respiratory protection to be used, and its modes of operation.
- The contaminant(s) to which the employee will be exposed, and related toxicity data.
- Tasks that the employee will perform while wearing the respirator.
- Visual and audio requirements associated with the task.
- Length of time that the user will wear the respiratory equipment.
- An estimation of the number of emergency or rescue situations.
- Length of time that the user may be required to spend in extreme environments.

The preceding information, obtained from plant management or a plant industrial hygienist, can be used to develop effective programs and procedures that are appropriate to specific operating locations and their conditions. At a minimum, the program should consist of the following:

1. Pre-employment or job change medical examination;
2. Routine periodic medical examination;
3. Examination on return to work following injury or prolonged illness; and
4. Medical records.

## PRE-EMPLOYMENT OR JOB
## CHANGE EXAMINATION

The pre-employment medical examination is a screening mechanism for respirator usage. At the end of this examination, the physician must be in a position to determine whether the worker is physically or mentally suitable for jobs requiring the use of respirators, and whether there are any particular jobs to which he should not be assigned or posts for which he is better suited. The examination should include the following parameters:

*History.*    The collection of data on his past occupational exposure, present or past respiratory disorders, and personal habits (smoking and hygiene) are two important elements.

The following is a list of questions that should be included on a questionnaire designed to identify these medical conditions:

1.  Have you ever been short of breath on exertion, such as (a) climbing one flight of stairs, (b) walking up a slight hill, or (c) walking with other people of your own age, at an ordinary pace on level ground?
2.  Have you ever had chest pains?
3.  Have you ever had asthma or emphysema?
4.  Do you frequently have difficulty breathing?
5.  Do you smoke?
6.  Have you ever had a heart attack or other heart condition?
7.  Do you have chronic skin problems of the face?
8.  Do you wear glasses or contact lenses?
9.  Do you have high blood pressure?
10. Do you know of any reason why you are not able to wear a respirator?

Any employee who has a past history of respiratory problems should be forbidden to wear a respirator that restricts inhalation and exhalation. For example, a person suffering from emphysema may be unable to breathe adequately against the additional resistance of a respirator. Similarly, if the user suffers an asthma attack, he would be likely to remove the respirator because he would be unable to breathe properly.

Details of previous workplace exposure must also be obtained during the initial medical examination. A record should be kept of jobs he has had since leaving school, on what conditions and for what duration, as well as any occupational accidents and diseases for which he may have been compensated. This is useful because many occupational diseases such as asbestosis, silicosis or occupational tumors often have a latent period.

*A General Physical Examination.*    In physical examinations, particular attention should be directed to physical and sensorial characteristics and those systems which may be affected by wearing respirators. The essential physical characteristics that should be noted are excessive weight, scars, hollow temples, very prominent cheekbones, deep skin creases, and lack of teeth or dentures, which may cause respirator facepiece-sealing problems and inability to use fingers or hands. Respirators such as gas masks, supplied-air respirators, and self-contained breathing apparatus require connection and disconnection of parts and manipulation of valves and fittings during use.

Persons with missing or disabled fingers may have difficulty in using these devices, particularly in an emergency when there may be no one present to assist them.

The significant sensorial characteristics to be noted are poor eyesight and poor hearing. These defects, if undetected, may increase the on-the-job risks involved in the use of certain types of respirators.

The correct functioning of the various systems of the body should also be checked. For example, presence of hernia can be aggravated by wearing/carrying respiratory equipment (SCBA). Temporary congestion caused by seasonal allergies (such as hayfever) may make it very unpleasant to work with a respirator on.

*Medical and Psychological Tests.*   Tests should be performed to examine the major systems. Pulmonary function tests should be undertaken in conjunction with x-rays and should include FVC and $FEV_1$. These tests will reveal respiratory insufficiency, including asthma, chronic bronchitis or emphysema. X-rays assist in determining the morphological state of the heart and its vascular pedicle. Blood and urine tests should be as extensive as necessary to detect anemia, hemophilia, and disorders resulting from occupational poisoning, or increased absorption of toxic substances (e.g., lead and mercury). Thus, medical tests must be general, as well as specific to the substance to which the employee will be exposed.

As stated earlier, some individuals may experience phobic sensations, or be anxious, due to a conscious appreciation of breathing. Unfortunately there is no diagnostic tool in use by which an occupational physician can screen these individuals. Hence psychological screening may become very subjective. However, when respirators are required to be used in emergency or rescue situations, the physician must take mental factors into consideration before recommending that psychologically affected individuals be allowed to work in situations where panic may endanger not only his life, but his co-workers' as well.


## PERIODIC EXAMINATION

Periodic examinations are traditionally designed for early detection and treatment of potentially dangerous disease, identifying risk factors, and prolonging life through risk-factor modification or early treatment.

For respirator users, there are some benefits of periodic examinations such as finding out what problems workers are having, answering their questions factually, educating workers on prudent work practices and respirator use, informing them of their exposure to toxicants and reassuring them through candid discussions. The periodic health evaluation ascertains that workers' capacities, as defined during the pre-employment examination, remain compatible with their occupation, as well as ensures that the work they carry out does not cause any additional disorder or lesion. Risk-factor intervention may appreciably improve the quality of life even though the length of life may not be increased. Workers who are successful in modifying harmful health practices usually derive impressive benefits. During these evaluations, much valuable health-experience information can be accumulated for future epidemiological studies. In addition, sudden temporary incapacitation or gradual deterioration of sensory facilities, alertness, or agility can also be detected.

The frequency of examinations will depend upon the age and health of workers and the risk factors associated with their jobs. For example, workers in excellent health with few or no risk factors and little exposure to toxic substances certainly need to be examined less frequently than those under multiple risks.

## EXAMINATION ON RETURN TO WORK AFTER AN INJURY OR PROLONGED ILLNESS

This evaluation should ensure that the worker whose work requires certain protective equipment is capable of resuming his usual work. Any changes in work capacity that may have been caused by the illness or accident should also be looked for, since permanent sequelae (physical handicaps) may make resumption of the former work impossible (occupational handicap). It then becomes necessary to reassign the worker.

An attempt should be made to find out if there is any connection between the injury and his job in order to improve preventive measures. It may be necessary for the physician to visit the workplace, investigate the environmental conditions and the precise nature of the substances used. Further questioning of the worker may reveal some valuable information regarding the working environment, the tempo of work, the efficiency of engineering controls and the use of various protective devices available to him.

If the worker does not use protective equipment, the reasons must be accurately determined by questioning him about all the operations he has to perform, their duration, their frequency and any technical changes that may have been introduced since he began his work. It may also be useful to find out his relationship with his supervisors, co-workers and subordinates.

## MEDICAL RECORDS

Medical records of a worker must be maintained for ready access to the documents relating to pre-employment examinations, periodic check-ups, the results of specialist, x-ray or laboratory tests, individual accident report forms and exposure records. These records should be maintained in a confidential file for use by the physician or nurse because, based on these confidential records, the physician concludes that a worker is fit, fit with limitations, or unfit to perform certain duties, and advises the employer accordingly, without revealing the details of personal records. Medical ethics require that complete observance of professional secrecy be maintained. In some countries, the examining physician is required by law to make certain disclosures of medical records to the worker or his union, and in some instances to judicial authorities. The necessary information can usually be given without impairing professional secrecy by limiting the disclosure of information to such facts as are absolutely essential.

## ACTIONS TO BE TAKEN ON MEDICAL INFORMATION

If a physician advises that a worker is fit with limitations, or unfit to wear respirators, the employer must act on this information. The precise action taken will depend on the professional advice of the physician. In many cases, there may be some choice as to the course of action taken, which can be worked out between the physician, the employer, and the worker.

If the results of clinical tests reach a critical level (e.g., .70 mg/L of blood lead) then the worker must be removed from exposure to the contaminant until results reach acceptable levels. High test results may be indicative of a lack of protection afforded by the use of respirators. A thorough investigation of the conditions of work and work practices of the worker must then be made.

The effectiveness of respirators under present conditions of work should also be examined. It is quite possible that conditions have changed significantly to warrant better respiratory protection, or better engineering controls, in order to reduce contaminant levels. Conversely, the results of clinical tests may not reach a critical level but the physician may still advise that a worker is fit with limitations, or unfit to wear respirators on the basis of other signs of adverse health effects.

The employer should adhere to the advice and information which the physician has provided, because it aids in evaluating and improving workplace controls. Although it may be necessary, in some cases, to provide more efficient respiratory protection, the best course of action is to reduce environmental contamination so that the worker does not have to be retrained for the use of new equipment.

## REFERENCE

1.  Withey, W.R. "Military Respirators: Physiological and Ergonomic Factors," *Respiratory Protection, Principles and Applications,* edited by B. Ballantyne and P.H. Schwabe, Chapman & Hall Ltd., London, 1981.

# 7

## *Criteria for a Respiratory Protection Program*

With all of the current legislation promulgating the use of engineering controls, work practices, and hygiene practices and facilities to control the exposure of a worker to a particular contaminant or to prevent atmospheric contaminants . . . as far as feasible by accepted engineering control measures, you may wonder why respiratory protection is needed. Regardless of any legislation, the responsibility of every employer should be to safeguard the health, safety and general well-being of their employees. In many cases this will involve the use of respirators.

Respirator use is only one alternative. As any alternative solution to a problem, its use should be determined by considering its risks, practicality, and cost-effectiveness. As a general rule of thumb, respirators should be used in:

1. Operations where environmental controls are being implemented or evaluated;
2. Operations where environmental controls are unavailable or cannot by themselves maintain an acceptable exposure level;
3. Operations involving constructions, maintenance, repair and decontamination where environmental controls may be unavailable or impracticable;
4. Emergencies where there is a health risk.

But using respirators opens a Pandora'a Box of questions regarding the protection we are getting, such as: What type of respirator should we use? Why are we using it? Is it the proper one? Does it fit? The questions go on. A respirator cannot be simply given to a worker with the expectation that it will provide total protection. It must be presented as part of a respiratory protection program. This chapter will highlight the necessary components of proper and effective programs. Previous chapters give more detailed explanations of individual components.

According to the current OSHA Standard, Section 1910.134, a formal respiratory protection equipment program is necessary when respirators are used in various manufacturing facilities. OSHA Standard 29CFR 1910.134(b) requirements for a minimally acceptable respiratory program are as follows:

(1) Written standard operating procedures governing the selection and use of respirators shall be established.

(2) Respirators shall be selected on the basis of hazards to which the worker is exposed.

(3) The user shall be instructed and trained in the proper use of respirators and their limitations.

(4) Where practicable, the respirators should be assigned to individual workers for their exclusive use.

(5) Respirators shall be regularly cleaned and disinfected. Those issued for the exclusive use of one worker should be cleaned after each day's use, or more often if necessary. Those used by more than one worker shall be thoroughly cleaned and disinfected after each use.

(6) Respirators shall be stored in a convenient, clean, and sanitary location.

(7) Respirators used routinely shall be inspected during cleaning. Worn or deteriorated parts shall be replaced. Respirators for emergency use such as self-contained devices shall be thoroughly inspected at least once a month and after each use.

(8) Appropriate surveillance of work-area conditions and degree of employee exposure or stress shall be maintained.

(9) There shall be regular inspection and evaluation to determine the continued effectiveness of the program.

(10) Persons should not be assigned to tasks requiring use of respirators unless it has been determined that they are physically able to perform the work and use the equipment. The local physician shall determine what health and physical conditions are pertinent. The respirator user's medical status should be reviewed periodically (for instance, annually).

(11) Approved or accepted respirators shall be used when they are available. The respirator furnished shall provide adequate respiratory protection against the particular hazard for which it is designed in accordance with standards established by competent authorities.

## THE RESPIRATORY PROTECTION PROGRAM

The first step in setting up a program is to assign a program administrator. The administrator, chosen on the basis of his training and experience, is solely responsible for all facets of the program. He must wear many hats in this position of coordinator, educator, supervisor, and consultant. The administrator must be fully aware of the hazards, posted areas, employee limitations, employee acceptance of respirators and he must also be familiar with all aspects of the business unit or organization.

The entire respiratory protection program should be outlined in written standard operating procedures. These procedures should be readily available to all people affected, especially the wearer, and cover:

1.  Identification of the hazard.
2.  Hazard assessment.
3.  Hazard control.
4.  Respirator selection.
5.  Respirator fit.
6.  Training program.
7.  Maintenance procedures.
8.  Medical surveillance.
9.  Program evaluation.

I will expand a little on each of these nine components.

### Identification of the Hazard

There are two basic conditions that need to be identified. The first is to identify the areas of the plant where there are problems. This involves in-depth consideration of the process, equipment, and the plant.

The second is to identify the type of hazard. For example, when we examine a particulate problem, dusts may be the only form of particulates you may be aware of. However, others exist as well, such as mists, fumes, spray, smoke, fog, smog, and radon daughters.

All particulate hazards require varying levels of protection. In general you can classify your problem into four main categories:

1.  Oxygen deficiency,
2.  Particulates,
3.  Gas/Vapors,
4.  A combination of all of these.

At least this general classification can narrow down the respirator selection procedure. However, as is the case with particulates, an in-depth look at the process and the chemistry involved within these categories is necessary to adequately define the level of protection needed.

### Hazard Assessment

A large part of the assessment stage is knowledge of the potential toxicity of the contaminant. Considerations include TLV, routes of entry and biological effects. The toxicity and behavior of individual chemicals will play a large part in the choice of a respirator.

In order to determine the exposure level, air samples of the workplace should be taken. Samples should represent work periods.

## Hazard Control

Problem areas identified by the assessment require effective engineering controls in order to reduce worker exposure to respiratory hazards. These include isolation, substitution, removing the source, and ventilation.

The purpose of the program is to protect the worker's respiratory system and the most effective way of doing this is by reducing exposure through technological improvements.

Where it is not practical for control procedures to be instituted, or during the time that controls are being installed, respiratory protection appropriate to the circumstances should be worn. Respirators should never be considered a substitute for engineered controls.

## Respirator Selection

Selection of the proper respirator is the most complex area of the program. We have seen that there are many different potential contaminants, as well as many different forms of contaminants, so it is not out of line to assume there are many different types of respirators as well.

A starting point in respirator selection is to look for an approval or certification label. Remember, however, that NIOSH does not have approval schedules for all contaminants, and in some instances the best product for the job may be unapproved.

As we have seen, there are a number of different types of respirators to select from. These include self-contained breathing apparati; supplied-air respirators; gas masks; dust, fume, and mist respirators; and chemical-cartridge or combination chemical-cartridge respirators. Selection of the proper respirator for a given situation requires considering: the nature of the hazard; characteristics of the hazardous operation or process; location of the hazardous area with respect to a safe area having respirable air; period of time in use; nature of the work; and the physical characteristics, functional capabilities, and limitations of various types of respirators. All factors and possibilities must be carefully examined by the administrator when selecting any respiratory device.

## Respirator Fit

The ability of a respirator to do the job depends particularly on the effectiveness of the respirator itself in a given environment and the proper use and fit of that respirator. It cannot be overemphasized that a proper fit must be obtained when respirators are worn. It is essential that the user know the capability of the respirator he is required to wear and the degree of protection he can reasonably expect from it. As we have discussed in Chapter 3, there are a number of factors which affect respirator fit. These are: design of the respirator; facial contours and facial hair; training, knowledge required for respirator selection; worker acceptance; and maintenance of respirators.

Respirators should be selected according to the characteristics of the hazard involved, the capabilities and limitations of the respirator and, most importantly, the ability of each respirator wearer to obtain a satisfactory fit.

Respirator fit, simply stated, is the ability of the device to interface with the wearer in such a manner as to prevent the workplace atmosphere from entering the worker's respiratory system. When the contaminated atmosphere penetrates the interface and enters the worker's breathing zone, exposure occurs. To effectively utilize respirators as a means of controlling airborne hazards, assessment and control must be made of the exposure resulting from a less than perfect fit.

There are a number of fit tests available. The two main types are the qualitative and quantitative fit tests. The qualitative or quantitative fit test should be used to determine the ability of each individual respirator wearer to obtain a satisfactory fit with a negative-pressure respirator. The results of these fit tests can be used to determine a Fit Factor.

The fit factor, as discussed in Chapter 3, is a measure of the degree of protection provided by the respirator to the wearer. The fit factor is a very important part of the decision system. It answers the question: does the respirator provide enough protection considering the concentration of the contaminant in the air which the worker is exposed to?

The results of a qualitative or quantitative respirator test should be used to select specific types, makes, and models of negative-pressure respirators for use by individual respirator wearers. The respirator-fitting test should be carried out at least annually for each wearer who uses a negative-pressure respirator.

## Training Program

This portion of a respiratory protection program is most often left out and it can least afford to be. Training brings the worker out of the dark. It answers a lot of his questions and reduces his skepticism. He will believe the respirator is to his benefit because he has participated in the program.

Training should be given to all people involved in the program especially supervisors, the person issuing respirators, and the wearer/worker.

Training should be carried out by a competent person and should include, as a minimum, the following items:

1. Instruction in the nature of the hazard, whether acute, chronic, or both, and an honest appraisal of what may happen if the proper device is not used.
2. An explanation of why engineering controls are not being applied or are not adequate, and what type of effort is being made to reduce or eliminate the need for respirators.
3. An explanation of why a particular type of respirator has been selected for a specific respiratory hazard.
4. Instruction and training in actual use (especially a respiratory protective device for emergency use) and close and frequent supervision to assure that it continues to be properly used.
5. Instruction in how to recognize and cope with emergency situations.
6. The user and his supervisor should be instructed and trained by competent instructors in the operation, limitations, and capabilities of the selected respirator(s).
7. Wearing instructions and training, including practical demonstrations, should be given to each respirator wearer and should cover:
   a. Donning, wearing, and removing the respirator,
   b. Adjusting the respirator so that it is properly fitted on the wearer and so that the respirator causes a minimum of discomfort to the wearer,
   c. Allowing the respirator wearer to wear the respirator in a safe atmosphere for an adequate period of time to ensure that the wearer is familiar with the operational characteristics of the respirator,
   d. Providing the respirator wearer with an opportunity to wear the respirator in a test atmosphere to demonstrate that the respirator provides protection to the wearer. A test atmosphere is any atmosphere in which the wearer can carry out activities simulating work movements, and respirator leakage or respirator malfunction can be detected by the wearer.
8. An explanation of how to maintain and store respirators.

If a good training program does not exist, the most obvious effect will be that workers will be exposed to an air contaminant. The result of this oversight, of course, could be fatal when a very toxic contaminant is being used.

## Maintenance Procedures

Each respirator used in the workplace should be properly maintained so that it may retain its original effectiveness. It is recommended that this portion of the respiratory protection program include procedures for:

1. Cleaning and sanitizing.
2. Inspection. After being cleaned and sanitized, each respirator should

be inspected and tested to determine if it is in proper working condition or whether it needs repair or removal from service.

3.  Repair and testing. When inspection indicates the respirator needs repair steps must be followed to ensure that proper repair and tests are carried out to confirm that the respirator is fully functional.
4.  Storage.
5.  Record keeping of maintenance, inspection, and testing procedures.

## Medical Surveillance

As necessary, biological monitoring of employees should be performed at regular intervals. Initially, the capability of the worker to wear a respirator must be determined through pulmonary-function testing. Periodically, usually annually, a physical examination should be performed.

## Program Evaluation

A program should never be stagnant. It should be evaluated annually and its procedures updated based on criticism and suggestions. The evaluation should consider:

1.  *Worker Acceptance.* The workers should be asked for comments on the respirator they are wearing regarding comfort, resistance to breathing, interference with vision, interference with communications, and confidence in respirator protection, etc. Bringing the wearer into the decision-making process will provide greater support to the program.
2.  *Inspections.* Frequent inspections should be conducted to ensure that each step in the program is being followed.
3.  *Appraisal of Protection Afforded.* Results of biological testing and results of area monitoring will indicate the degree of effectiveness of the program.

The findings of the respirator evaluation should be documented, and concrete target dates listed to implement corrective action.

In summary, in order to comply with the OSHA standard and other countries' occupational health and safety legislation and to provide the worker with adequate respiratory protection, a respiratory protection program must be established. This chapter summarizes the necessary components of this program. Some facilities may require an extensive program while others may need only a minimum program. Manufacturing plants should require only one respirator program, while pilot plants or laboratories may require several, depending on the administration involved. Each facility should determine its current respirator usage and projected needs. If it is determined

Table 7.1  Respiratory protection program written format

PROGRAM

I. Introduction

In the control of those occupational diseases caused by breathing air contaminated with gases or aerosols, the primary objective is to prevent harmful exposures. This is accomplished as far as feasible by accepted engineering control measures – (for example, general and local ventilation, enclosure or isolation, and substitution of less hazardous processes or materials). When effective engineering controls are not feasible, or while they are being instituted, appropriate respirators may be required.

II. Purpose and Scope

The practices and procedures described here constitute the program under which respirators are effectively utilized at _____

III. Responsibility

A. _____ is the respirator program coordinator. He is responsible for:

1. Provision of appropriate respirators.

2. Implementing training and instruction programs.

3. Administering the overall program.

INSTRUCTIONS

Underlined statements or blanks are to be filled in by the plant to fit the program to the specific needs of the plant or area where respirators are used. The name of the plant or area goes here.

The title of one individual in the plant should be named here as overall coordinator of the respirator program. This person might be the plant engineer, the plant safety coordinator, plant superintendent, or a process engineer.

INSTRUCTIONS

B. Supervisory personnel are responsible for:

1. Ensuring that respirators are available as needed.

2. Ensuring that employees wear respirators as required.

3. Inspection of respirators on a regular schedule.

C. The employee is responsible for:

1. Using the respirator supplied to him/her in accordance with instructions and training.

2. Cleaning, disinfecting, inspecting and storing his/her respirator.

3. Reporting a respirator malfunction to supervision.

D. The _____ is responsible for:

1. Ensuring that the standards include the requirement for respirator use where necessary.

The employee's responsibility here is very important. Effective training and supervision will be essential. Some plants with large respirator programs may want to assign a specific individual to clean and inspect all the respirators. If this is the case, this paragraph may be rewritten to reflect the actual situation. The employee should, however, always inspect his respirator before use.

Fill in the first blank in this paragraph with the title of the person who will review the process description used in your plant and determine at what point the respiratory protection equipment should be utilized. (This could be the process engineer, respirator program coordinator, etc.)

The second blank in this paragraph refers to the name given to the process description or operating standard used in your plant. Please fill in the appropriate term.

Table 7.1   (*continued*)

| | INSTRUCTIONS |
|---|---|
| E.   Industrial Hygiene Services is responsible for: | Surveillance of the work area conditions is essential to an effective respirator program. Air sampling and industrial hygiene surveys are needed to determine the proper application and safety of respirator use. |
| 1. Technical assistance in determining the need for respirators and in the selection of appropriate types. | |
| 2. Providing surveillance of work area conditions. | |
| 3. Periodically evaluating the respirator program. | |
| 4. Providing educational materials to be used in employee training. | |
| F.   Safety is responsible for: | The coordinator of the respirator program should discuss with his Safety Engineer the need for emergency respirators. The need will depend on the type of potential hazards that may be present within the plant. |
| 1. Technical assistance in the selection of respirators for use in emergency reentry situations and the training and instructions necessary for their use. | |

IV. Respirator Selection

Respirators are selected by the respirator program coordinator and Industrial Hygiene Services. This choice is based on the physical, chemical and physiological properties of the air contaminant and on the concentration likely to be encountered. The quality of fit and the nature of the work being done also affect the choice of respirators. The capability of the respirators chosen is determined from appropriate governmental approvals, manufacturers' tests and plant experience with the respirators.

V. Distribution

Respirators are issued to individuals whenever possible. Each respirator which is individually assigned is identified in a way that does not interfere with its performance.

VI. Inspection and Maintenance

Respirators are properly maintained to retain their original effectiveness by: periodic inspection, repair, cleaning and proper storage.

A. Inspection

1. All respirators are inspected routinely by the user before and after each use and after cleaning, to check condition of face piece, head bands, valves and hoses; and canister, filter or cartridge fit.

2. The foreman or supervisor inspects all respirators at least once per month.

3. Respirators maintained for emergency use are tagged noting the date of inspection, and the initials of the person doing the inspection. A log indicating these inspections is maintained in the plant office.

This includes those respirators which are not used routinely, as well as those which are. You may wish to establish a method of recording this inspection. If so, it should be indicated at this point in the program.

These tags are available and can be supplied to you for this purpose; or, you can develop your own tag system.

Table 7.1 *(continued)*

| | INSTRUCTIONS |
|---|---|
| B. Maintenance | |
| Respirators which do not pass inspections are replaced or repaired immediately. Repair of the respirator by the user is limited to changing canisters, cartridges, filters and head straps. All other replacements or repairs are performed by _____, an experienced person with parts designed for the respirator. No attempt is made to replace components, or make adjustments, modifications or repairs beyond the manufacturer's recommendations. | The "experienced person" mentioned here should be a designated technician who is trained or experienced in the repair of all respirators used. If he has a title you may wish to substitute it here. |
| VII. Cleaning | |
| Individually assigned respirators are cleaned and disinfected as frequently as necessary to insure that proper protection is provided for the wearer. Respirators not individually assigned and those for emergency use are cleaned and disinfected after each use. | |
| The following procedure is used for cleaning and disinfecting respirators: | |
| A. Filters, cartridges, or canisters are removed before washing the respirator and discarded as necessary. | |
| B. Respirators are washed in a detergent solution, rinsed in clean water and allowed to dry in a clean area. A brush is used to scrub the respirator to remove adhering dirt. | |

VIII. Storage

After inspection, cleaning and necessary repairs, respirators are stored to protect against dust, sunlight, heat, extreme heat, extreme cold, excessive moisture, or damaging chemicals.

IX. Training

Every employee who may have to wear a respirator is trained in the proper use of the respirator. Both the employee and his supervisor receive this training. This training includes:

A. Description of the respirators.

B. Intended use and limitations of the respirator.

C. Proper wearing, adjustment, and testing for fit.

D. Cleaning and storage methods.

E. Inspection and maintenance procedures.

This training is repeated as necessary, at least annually, to ensure that employees remain familiar with the proper use of respiratory protection. The training program is evaluated at least annually by the program coordinator to determine its continued effectiveness.

INSTRUCTIONS

It is recommended that respirators be stored in plastic bags or the original cartons and placed in specially designated cabinets or lockers with other protective equipment. Under most conditions it is not advisable to store a respirator in a tool box or in the open. Cartridges or canisters and masks equipped with these components should be sealed in plastic bags to preserve their effectiveness. Improper storage will usually result in reduced service life and added cost.

Training program materials for respirator use will be made available by Industrial Hygiene Services. Training and reference materials may be attached to the respirator program as additional Appendices.

Table 7.1 *(continued)*

X. Records

The following records are maintained by:

A. The number and types of respirators in use.

B. A record of employee training programs.

C. Inspection and maintenance reports.

D. Medical certification that the employee is capable of wearing a respirator under his given work conditions.

INSTRUCTIONS

Record keeping personnel are to be determined by the plant. Please fill in the title of the individual selected. The respirator program coordinator is suggested.

OSHA regulations require a medical determination that an individual required to use a respirator must be physically able to perform the work and use the equipment.

Signed: _____  Respirator Program Coordinator

Approved: _____  Plant Manager

_____  Industrial Hygiene Services

that respirators are not required at a facility, then a program is not necessary. A program coordinator should be selected in the plant to oversee the in-house development of the basic program.

Initially, the setting up of an effective respiratory protective program will require a good deal of time and energy, but once established it will provide the company and employees with a concise and accurate step in the direction of better health and safety.

Table 7.1 is a sample respiratory protection program that can be used as a guideline in developing your program.

# 8

## *Industrial Applications: Case Studies*

This chapter contains examples of problems associated with industrial use of respirators. These examples are based on our experiences and those of others over a period of many years. In many cases, firsthand information was obtained by actually visiting a variety of workplaces where respiratory hazards exist. We observed that the proper use of respirators is difficult to achieve because of:

1.  The lack of proper training programs, including information on limitations associated with respirator use;
2.  The lack of proper inspection and administration;
3.  The user being reluctant to accept a particular respirator due to additional stress that it may cause, including interference with his ability to see, his freedom to move, and his ability to communicate;
4.  The lack of testing facilities on-site resulting in incorrect selection and improper fitting of respirators;
5.  The lack of proper maintenance and care program, resulting in improper functioning and reduced efficiency of the respirator;
6.  A lack of understanding of NIOSH approval criteria;
7.  Confusion regarding the use of respirators in conjunction with engineering controls;
8.  The problems associated with specific terminologies used by experts.

This chapter attempts to illustrate the most commonly occurring misuses and excuses due to the above problems.

### LACK OF TRAINING, INCLUDING INFORMATION ON LIMITATIONS

#### A Case Study: Oxygen Deficiency

A workman entered a sewer manhole located in a street just outside a brewery. After a few minutes, he felt tired and weak. He tried to climb out of the manhole, but collapsed. A worker in the brewery, seeing this, rushed over with a respirator. The workman's helper grabbed an immediately available respirator, put it on, and proceeded into the manhole. Within a few minutes, he too passed out. When the two men were finally rescued by the Fire Department, they were both dead.

This clearly illustrates the hazard of selecting improper respirators. In this case, carbon dioxide from the brewery had entered the sewer and displaced the air. The two men died from a deficiency of oxygen; as the respirator used by the rescuer was designed to remove ammonia from air it could not supply oxygen for breathing.

The following recommendations were made to prevent this occurrence in the future:

1. Do not permit entry into an enclosed space without first checking its oxygen content. Do not enter any atmosphere with less than 19.5% oxygen without appropriate respiratory protection. When there is a question concerning the oxygen content of the atmosphere, an oxygen-deficiency measurement should be made.
2. Prior to entry, inform the individuals making the entry as to what hazards will be encountered.
3. If the area is oxygen-deficient, only a self-contained breathing apparatus should be used.
4. The individual making the entry must wear a life-line controlled by an individual outside the oxygen-deficient atmosphere. He must also wear self-contained breathing equipment and maintain visual contact with the individual in the oxygen-deficient atmosphere at all times. A third individual, also wearing self-contained breathing equipment, must also be standing by to provide aid if necessary.
5. A training program must be provided giving adequate instruction on the limitation of equipment.

## LACK OF INSPECTION AND ADMINISTRATION

### A Case Study: Hydrocarbon Vapor Exposure

A workman who entered an underground fuel oil tank to check the amount of sludge at the bottom of the tank was wearing a World War II gas mask. Shortly after entering the tank, he passed out. A second man, also wearing a World War II gas mask, entered the tank to rescue his fellow worker. He attached a rope to the unconscious man and then collapsed face down in the oil and sludge, tearing the air hose from his mask in the fall. The first man was pulled from the tank and recovered quickly. Because of the position of the rescuer after collapsing, he aspirated considerable oil and sludge, and died twelve hours after being pulled from the tank.

In this case, a high concentration of hydrocarbon vapors, sufficient to cause narcosis, was present in the tank. A World War II gas mask was originally designed to remove war gases from air, and it is not certain whether it is capable of removing hydrocarbons.

The following recommendations were made for the future:

1. A standard procedure must be developed to include all information necessary for the safe use of respirators in routine or emergency situations.
2. Possible emergency uses should be anticipated and recorded in writing.
3. The correct respirator for each job must be specified by a qualified individual supervising the program.
4. The rescuer or standby man must be equipped with a self-contained breathing apparatus.
5. Frequent, random inspections must be conducted by a trained individual to ¬ssure that respirators are properly selected, used, cleaned, and maintained.

## LACK OF MAINTENANCE

### A Case Study: Dust Exposure

During one of our surveys, a worker was found wearing a respirator with the exhalation valve jammed in the open position. Thus, dust was allowed to leak through the respirator. The obvious need for corrective maintenance was pointed out to the employee with the following recommendation:

1. All respirators must be inspected for defects (including a leak check), cleaning and disinfecting, repair and storage.
2. All respirators must be inspected before and after each use, and on a routine basis.
3. If the respirator is not used routinely and stored between uses, it must be inspected at least once every month and kept in good working condition.
4. When inspecting a respirator, all connections must be tight and the facepiece, headbands, valves and connecting tubes must be in proper working order.
5. Whenever respirators are inspected, tested, and repaired, the work must be performed by trained individuals.
6. Instruction should be provided to the trainee regarding how to determine if a respirator is in good operating condition.

## IMPROPER SELECTION OF RESPIRATOR

### A Case Study: Vapor Degreaser

The operation of a fully enclosed trichloroethylene vapor degreaser was restricted by parts falling into and covering the heating elements. The degreaser was shut down at 9:00 a.m. and by 11:00 a.m. the degreaser had been drained and a compressed air-line set up to blow out the enclosure. In addition, an exhaust fan at the discharge end of the degreaser was turned on.

At about 11:45 a.m. a maintenance worker climbed down a ladder into the degreaser to recover fallen parts. He was wearing a cartridge-type respirator. A second man was posted on a platform above the degreaser. The first man collapsed in the degreaser. The second man called for help and climbed down into the degreaser to rescue his pal. He also collapsed. Before the event was finished, six other fellow workers had entered the degreaser, and three firemen were called to the scene. All except one fireman were to some extent overcome by the solvent vapors. The firemen were wearing SCBA.

There was an inch or so of solvent left in the degreaser after draining, but the surface for evaporation is more important than the total volume of fluid. In this case, the air above the surface could be saturated with trichloroethylene (as high as 9.78%). Because of the heavy vapor, there would be little tendency for the air moving system to remove vapors.

A cartridge-type respirator is suitable for not more than 0.1% vapor. A gas mask could be adequate for 2% vapor, but only an air-line respirator or self-contained air-supplied respirator would have been suitable in this case.

The following recommendations were made:

1.  Before entering an atmosphere, air samples must be taken to ensure the compatibility of the atmosphere with the use of an available respirator.
2.  Samples must be taken and analyzed by a qualified hygienist.
3.  The selection of a respirator must be made by an individual who is qualified to do so.
4.  The user must be made aware that the cartridge cannot be used in atmospheres containing concentrations greater than those stated on the cartridge.
5.  Standby men or rescuers must always use SCBA.

## RELUCTANCE TO USE A RESPIRATOR

### A Case Study: Hydrogen Sulfide Exposure

Three men were pumping the contents from a tan-yard vat when the pump inlet plugged. One man entered the vat to unplug the line and passed out. A second man entered to recover the first victim and he also passed out. A third man entered to assist and felt quite dizzy, but he was able to crawl from the vat using a ladder. Within a few minutes he had help. He warned a fourth man not to enter the tank, but the man entered anyway, and he also passed out. With further help, the three bodies were removed, but none of them could be resuscitated.

An investigation revealed that proper respirators were available on-site, but none of the men bothered to use them. The vat had not been in use for about four years. The sludge from the vat, when aerated, released up to 4 mg./liter air (2700 ppm.) hydrogen sulfide. The men, by disturbing the sludge, released heavy concentrations of hydrogen sulfide.

## A Case Study: Isocyanate Exposure

In an autobody shop, all painters engaged in the spray-painting of cars with polyurethane paints were using half-masks with charcoal filters. They were all found to be sensitized against isocyanates.

Investigation revealed that, although supplied-air respirators were available, the painters did not like using them due to the inconvenience. They tended to use filtering devices, typically half-masks.

In the two cases cited above, the following recommendations were made:

1. All workers must be educated regarding the benefits of wearing respirators when required.
2. The toxic materials as well as their expected concentration in each operation should be identified. Also, the possible effect on the body of long or short-term exposure (if the respirator is not worn), and what protection the respirator will provide, should also be explained.
3. The worker must be taught to read the label on the filter cartridge to be sure that the proper filter is being used for the contaminant present.
4. Positive and firm enforcement of respirator usage must be followed.
5. Records of employees' negligence should be kept.

## LACK OF TESTING FACILITIES ON-SITE

### A Case Study: Chlorine Exposure

In a plant producing chlorine gas, individual exposures to chlorine were usually less than 1 ppm. time-weighted average. Occasionally, spills would occur and for these emergency situations, the employees were provided with half-face chemical-cartridge respirators for their escape. It was found that, although the majority of employees effectively utilized their respirators for safe evacuation, a few employees still required medical treatment.

Investigations revealed that the major cause for the trouble was poor facepiece-to-face seal due to facial hair and facial features. Since there were no facilities available on-site for either qualitative or quantitative fit tests, it was virtually impossible to determine who needed better protection, i.e., full-face mask, rather than half-face mask.

The following suggestions were made:

1.  Each worker should be provided with a respirator which will provide him with the same level of protection that his fellow employees are receiving.
2.  Qualitative fit tests must be done for each respirator/wearer combination to determine facepiece to face-seal leakage.
3.  Positive and negative fit tests should be performed by the wearer before entering a contaminated atmosphere.
4.  If the leakage is considerable, due to facial features, a full-face mask respirator must be used for a better seal.
5.  Each person who wears a respirator should be checked for fit at least annually by a qualified individual. Aging, gains or losses in weight, or any of a number of other factors can affect the fit of a particular mask, and may make necessary a change to another brand.

## MISINTERPRETATION OF NIOSH TESTING AND APPROVAL CRITERIA

### A Case Study: Removal of Insulation Containing Asbestos[1]

In this case, insulation containing asbestos was being removed from steel beams. Since the worksite was not permanent, local or general ventilation was not feasible. Respirators were the only means available to control the exposure to dust. A visit to the site revealed that the workers engaged in removing insulation were wearing non-approved disposable dust respirators, and the tradesmen in the area were not wearing any respirators.

During our visit, it was observed that tradesmen not wearing respirators grabbed the first available respirator lying around the job site and put it on.

### A Case Study: Discrepancy in NIOSH Approvals

In an asbestos removal job the contractor had supplied his workers with the type of respirators listed under NIOSH TC-21C type S. On our visit, we recommended that instead of type S, type A should be used to better protect the employees. The contractor objected to our recommendation because, in his opinion, there was no difference between type A and type S.

The NIOSH Certified Equipment List (NCEL) [2] describes A-type as "designed as respiratory protection against asbestos-containing dusts and mists," and S-type as "designed as respiratory protection against pneumoconiosis and fibrosis-producing dusts, or dusts and mists." Considering the wording used to specify each protection type, selection of an A-type is the obvious choice of worker protection for asbestos environments. However, since asbestos is a pneumoconiosis-producing dust, selection of S-type also appears to be appropriate according to NIOSH. Unfortunately, the published lists of certified equipment by NIOSH do not clarify these apparent discrepancies and the respirator manufacturers tend to highlight these vague areas in their advertising. For example, the container of one type of single-use respirator states, "NIOSH/MSA approved for dusts and mists (including lead and asbestos)." The respirator in question has an approval under the S category. It is plain to see that the manufacturer has designed the package label to take the broader meaning of pneumoconiosis-producing dusts, i.e., including asbestos. The person selecting a respirator would not be able to verify the manufacturer's claim(s) using the current NCEL. An experienced and trained person with industrial hygiene experience will, in most cases, opt for more stringent protection and select the A-type. However, an ordinary respirator selector would tend to read the label and select a respirator on this basis without further verifying the details. A compliance officer from the Government would also invariably consider the S-type as complying with the requirement of controlling workers' exposure to asbestos.

The following recommendations were made:

1. The contractor should provide respirators that are appropriate, under the circumstances, for the type and concentration of airborne asbestos.
2. Ideally, all dust exposures should be thoroughly evaluated by air sampling before respiratory protection is prescribed. In the construction industry, this is not always possible since the jobsite changes so frequently that by the time the sampling is done and results are available, the job is finished. In situations such as this, when adequate information is not readily available, it must be assumed that the greatest hazard possible is present, and consequently, the use of 'A' type respirators listed with NCEL should be made mandatory.
3. A respirator which is not approved by NIOSH or an equivalent agency is considered to be non-approved. It should not be used for protection against asbestos under any circumstances.
4. When it is not possible to provide adequate engineering controls for dust-producing operations, it is imperative that any persons coming into the area wear approved respirators. The fact that people (i.e., other tradesmen, supervisors) are not directly involved in the production of dust, or may only be in the area for a short period of time, does not absolve them from the need to be protected from the dust by wearing a proper respirator.

5.  Respirators lying around the job site gathering dust should never be used by any person in the area for the obvious reason that one may inhale an excessive amount of dust in the first breath.


## ENGINEERING CONTROLS VS. RESPIRATORS

### A Case Study: Abrasive Blasting

In one company, abrasive blasting using silica sand was used to clean metal parts in a booth ventilated according to the ACGIH *Ventilation Manual* criteria[3]. Both the blaster and his helper were wearing air-purifying respirators. When asked to change to air-supplied respirators, the employer maintained that ventilation had been provided to control the dust being produced and the respirators had been provided only as an extra precautionary measure. It was therefore unreasonable to ask for air-supplied respirators.

In order to convince the employer, several 8-hour personal samples for silica were taken. The results were 10 to 50 times the standard of 0.1 mg./m$^3$.

The following recommendation was made:

1.  For abrasive blasting operations involving silica sand, ventilation in the blasting booth is provided merely to keep the dust down for visibility purposes. Hence, air-supplied respirators must be used to protect the workers from the siliceous dust generated.


### A Case Study: Paint Sprayers

In an assembly plant for heavy-duty trucks, spray-painting was done using compressed air-spray guns in five spray booths. Paints containing lead were used in all the spray booths. In one of these booths, which happened to be the largest, truck cabs were spray-painted by two painters. The booth was equipped with a down-draft, waterwash-type ventilation system, as well as air curtains at the entry/exit openings of the booth. The results of ventilation measurements proved to be in accordance with the recommended design criteria for spray-paint booths outlined in the ACGIH *Ventilation Manual*[3]. No respirators were deemed necessary for the sprayers.

During routine monitoring of employees' exposures, it was discovered that the lead-air monitoring results were above the short-term exposure limit (STEL). The employer was asked to provide adequate respirators to the sprayers. The sprayers refused to wear them, alleging that "a properly designed ventilation spray-booth should not require use of respirators by spray painters." The following counter argument persuaded the sprayers to wear the proper respirators:

In large paint booths, there are too many variables which can affect the airborne concentrations during painting, so it isn't safe to rely on ventilation alone. Differences in paint viscosity and compressed air pressure of the spray gun may increase the amount of paint deflected into the air due to *bounceback* or the painter may need to stand upstream of the exhaust ventilation in order to paint a certain area of the truck. When there is more than one sprayer in the booth, spraying onto the same object from different directions may cause excessive aerosol generation into another's breathing zone before ventilation takes effect. Hence, a respirator is the only means of assuring the painter of the lowest practical exposure.

The following recommendations were made:

1.   In addition to the ventilation provided for the large paint-booths, the sprayers should be required to wear approved respirators, even if the ventilation meets the recommended criteria.
2.   Sprayers' exposures must be regularly monitored to determine the efficiency of respirators being used.

## A Case Study: Asbestos/Silica Handling

A large company was involved in dumping, mixing and bagging a powdered product which contained a small percentage of asbestos and silica. A large amount of money was spent to install adequate local mechanical exhaust at each dust-producing operation. The company was very concerned about the hazards of exposure to dust and thus, as an extra measure of protection, tried to force all workers to wear respirators even though adequate ventilation was provided. The employees complained to a Government authority that they were being subjected to unnecessary work stress.

An investigation revealed that the ventilation provided was more than adequate to protect the workers from asbestos and silica exposure. The results of a sampling were 1/5th to 1/10th the recommended standards.

The following recommendations were made:

1.   The purpose of providing engineering controls should be to protect the worker from respiratory hazards and thus make wearing respirators unnecessary.
2.   In the event that engineering methods of control are not adequate, respirators should be worn until improvements are made.
3.   As a last resort, if controls are not adequate and further improvements are not feasible, then the use of respirators may also be necessary.

## PROBLEMS ASSOCIATED WITH
## AIR-LINE RESPIRATORS

### A Case Study: Asbestos Exposure[4]

In a plant producing brake lining, a significant exposure to asbestos was occurring at the operation where dry mix containing asbestos was hand-scooped from a tote box into a preform press hopper. Although the hopper was ventilated in a limited way, the tote box was unventilated and considerable dust was produced each time the operator transferred a portion of the mix. Although work practices definitely affected the worker's exposure, it was found that no matter how carefully the operator worked, his exposure was always above the legal standard.

As an interim measure, until improvements in ventilation and possible process changes were implemented, the operator was required to wear a respirator. The company felt that a continuous air-flow helmet would give adequate protection.

Since two motor skids were used to move metal tote boxes into and out of the area, it was decided that the airline hose could not be allowed to drag along the floor. Thus, a clothesline was installed above the hoppers and the airline was coiled around this to prevent it from contacting the floor.

While this system seemed good in theory, a visit to the plant revealed a number of problems that were preventing the operator from receiving the protection he theoretically should have.

The first problem was that the airline became badly tangled. This resulted in the operators having to tug and pull on the line. Thus, the respirator was a hindrance to him and, occasionally, the operator would remove the helmet.

The second problem was that because of tangling and pulling, the airline was worn in places and minor leaks resulted. This reduced the flow of air to the helmet and subsequently reduced respiratory protection.

Third, although the helmets were provided with clear visors, it was common to see the visors flipped up.

While continuous-flow airline helmets can offer a high degree of protection, the abuses observed prevented the operators from receiving adequate protection. The airline hose was too much of an inconvenience since it had to be kept off of the floor.

Due to the abuses and limitations of the airline respirator in this situation, the company switched over to a powered air-purifying respirator which provided adequate protection.

The following recommendations were made:

1.  Airline respirators suffer from serious limitations due to the long air hoses connected to them, hence, before selecting an airline respirator,

other alternatives must be considered. It is quite possible that the airline respirators provide too much protection for the job intended.

2. The air flow inside the helmet must be regularly checked to detect reduction in airflow resulting from kinks or other obstructions in the air-supply line.

## PROBLEMS ASSOCIATED WITH FACIAL HAIR

### A Case Study: Beards

A bearded firefighter using a demand-type SCBA was asked by his employer to shave off his beard in order to provide a good face seal. The firefighter complained to the Human Rights Commission alleging that it was an invasion of his personal and religious rights to be told that he could not have facial hair.

A ruling was made that the employer was right in asking the employee to remove his facial hair for the purpose of safety.

Our recommendation was that:

1. If a firefighter objects to removing his facial hair due to personal or religious reasons, then only pressure-demand SCBA should be provided to protect him from toxic contaminants. This is because a demand-type SCBA maintains negative pressure in the facepiece, thus increasing the risk of leakage.
2. Although the pressure-demand SCBA will likely give adequate protection, the service-life of an air tank may be reduced from 30 minutes to 20-25 minutes due to outward leaks caused by a beard.

## REFERENCES

1. Rajhans, G.S., Brown, D.A., "Employee Education—Management Support Can Halt Respirator Abuse," *Occupational Health and Safety,* July/August, 1978; 30–34.
2. "Supplement to the NIOSH Certified Equipment List," DHHS (NIOSH) Publication No. 82-106, Cincinnati (October 1981).
3. *Industrial Ventilation—A Manual of Recommended Practice,* American Conference of Governmental Industrial Hygienists, 17th ed., Cincinnati (1982).
4. Brown, D.A., "Respiratory Protection," *Occupational Health in Ontario,* Vol. No. 4, October, 1981; 179–190.

# 9

---

# *Research Needs*

---

Respirators have been around for hundreds and hundreds of years. From the early Greek and Roman times, through the middle ages and the industrial revolution and even today, respirators are used by man to help protect his health. We have come a long way from the time when animal bladders and sponges were used to prevent the inhalation of harmful materials.

Within the last fifty years respiratory protection has changed drastically. Recent advancements have been numerous. These advancements include applications of technology to provide enhanced particulate filtration, the use of different chemical sorbents for more efficient air cleaning, the design of new ways to provide powered air-purifying respirators, qualitative and quantitative face fit techniques, respirator training programs, and the testing and certification of existing respirators.

Has the development of respiratory protection gone as far as it can? We and others do not feel that this is the case. This chapter deals with the future research needs in the field of respiratory protection.

There are two aspects of respiratory protection that must be considered when we speak of any development. These are the respirator component and the wearer component of the wearer-respirator interface. You could develop the most fantastic respirator that protects against all toxic materials in today's workplace, but if the worker will not wear it, for whatever reason, then what good is it? The wearer component of this two component interface is critical in any future work in this field. In the past most, if not all, research has dealt with the respirator. It is now time to include the wearer's needs, feelings and requirements in our research. This chapter will look at both components and the need for tying the two together in future research.

Researchers working on a new respirator must be able to answer a number of questions, some of which are:

1. What is to be protected against?
2. What are the chemical and physical properties of the contaminant?
3. How does the contaminant exist in areas of use?
4. Where will the respirator be used?
5. What other contaminants are also present?
6. How long must the respirator last?

7.  Is there a P.E.L.? If so, what is it?
8.  What is the odor threshold?
9.  Does NIOSH or another certification agency have an approval schedule for this respirator?
10. If so, what are the NIOSH tests?
11. What is the potential market?
12. Can a better respirator be designed, manufactured and marketed successfully?

Not all of these questions can be answered easily, but they must be if the research is to be successful and useful.

The emphasis of most occupational health and safety legislation in the Western World is on the control of the workplace environment through engineering and administration controls, rather than the use of personnel-protective equipment. The use of respiratory protection is considered to be an interim method to help protect the worker until the process can be changed, the hazardous material is substituted, the ventilation system is installed, etc.

Engineering controls have been slow in implementation, especially in times of "tight money." Because of the reluctance to spend a lot of money on using engineering to rid the workplace of hazards, respirators are relied on heavily. We see this reliance on the use of respirators continuing into the near future and possibly beyond. This then creates concern for the adequacy of respiratory protection and thus generates an increased emphasis on respirator research and development. Answers must be found in the future for questions of today.

One of the problems with any type of respiratory protection is that no one is willing to wear a respirator for an extended period of time. As soon as one has to wear a respirator, problems occur: it is hard to breathe through; it is too hot; it is too heavy; it hurts; I can't see or talk with it on; etc. Are these complaints real or not? It is not important to answer this question. The important point is to realize that there are psychological problems with the wearer associated with the use of respiratory equipment. This is the wearer component of that wearer-respirator interface which we mentioned earlier. There has been very limited research to date done on the psychological aspects of wearing a respirator.

In September 1983 W.P. Morgan published a review article on the psychological problems associated with the use of respirators in the *American Industrial Hygiene Association Journal* [1]. Wearer comfort seems to be the primary criteria in respirator selection by the wearer. It seems that most people experience distress when wearing a respirator. The amount of distress seems to be dependent on a number of factors such as type of facepiece, ability to see, ability to breathe easily, and ease of communication. Comfort can mean different things to different people. Comfort characteristics as they relate to a respirator are weight, breathing resistance, face seal, heat and moisture. Types of respirators that can be successfully worn for any extended period of time seem to be those that have addressed these comfort characteristics. They are:

1. Lightweight.
2. Low pressure drop so breathing resistance is as low as possible but filtering efficiency is adequate.
3. The respirator is simple to put on.
4. Face seal is easy to check.
5. Face seal is good but not tight enough to hurt.
6. Temperature and moisture build-up inside the respirator are minimal.

More research is needed by the respirator manufacturers to address these comfort characteristics and meet the wearer's requirements as far as comfort is concerned.

Morgan's review article points out that psychological problems seem to be associated with feelings of claustrophobia and the added distress of sweat and pressure on the skin. Also he points out that it appears that psychometric performance (i.e., information processing and decision making) of the wearer seems to be imposed by the use of a respirator. More research into this area is needed. One of Morgan's findings was that all existing data on the psychological aspects of wearing respiratory protection was based upon laboratory experiments involving healthy, young males who had volunteered to participate in the studies. There have been attempts to extend the findings to generalize the total workforce population. Extensive research is needed into the psychological aspects of wearing respiratory protection in actual workplace conditions.

If more extensive studies were carried out on the physiological and psychological stresses experienced by the respirator wearer more information would be made available to the manufacturer as to the necessary performance criteria that the wearer would require in order to wear an acceptable (to the wearer) respirator for the necessary extended periods of time in order to protect his health. Also the medical profession would have more data available to them which would permit them to establish better medical limitations for respirator wearers.

In the United States NIOSH certifies respirators. NIOSH approval is accepted by other occupational health and safety jurisdictions, such as Canada where there is no respirator certification program as the standard requirement for respirator use. The United States is not the only country with a respirator certification program. There are others such as Germany, Great Britain and Japan, to name a few. In several recent articles by Ryan et al in the *American Industrial Hygiene Association Journal,* the respirator certification programs of many of the other countries have been summarized [2–4].

The primary function of any respirator certification program is to set criteria which will ensure that a minimum level of performance is met by a particular respirator. Second, the certification program should provide information on the proper conditions for usage and spell out any limitations of the respirator. Does this happen? We feel that these objectives are not totally met. There is a need for further research and work in the area of respirator certification programs.

Performance criteria under the respiratory certification programs summarized by Ryan et al for particulate respirators show that the test aerosol varies from sodium chloride used in Germany and others to silica used by NIOSH [2]. Liquid aerosols are also used by many countries, while Germany uses paraffin oil and several others use silica mist. Not all countries test respiratory equipment with both solid and liquid aerosols. More research is needed to determine what the difference is in filter efficiencies using solid and liquid aerosols. Both tests should be required until more specific data are collected to determine how they relate to respirator-filtering capability.

Very little is known about the effect of relative humidity on the filter efficiency of particulate-type respirators. This should be determined in order to decide whether high-relative-humidity test conditions should be incorporated into respirator certification programs.

According to Ryan et al certification standards should incorporate more specific procedures and types of apparatus in the tests [2]. Also there is too much variety in testing methods and one set of internationally agreed upon test procedures should be incorporated into all respirator certification programs.

The efficiency of an absorbent in filtering organic vapors depends on a number of variables such as a particular compound being removed, temperature, humidity, and flow rate through the absorbing material. Because of these effects, an organic-vapor respirator, whether canister or cartridge type, will have different absorption capabilities for different organic vapors. Yet all countries that have respirator certification programs use only carbon tetrachloride to test organic vapor respirators [3]. How well carbon tetrachloride predicts the protection capabilities of respirators against other organic vapors is a question that must be addressed through extensive research and data gathering.

Conditions used in respirator certification programs of all countries were found not to be representative of the actual environment that the gas/vapor respirators are used in [3]. Test concentrations are usually well in excess of those found in the workplace, temperature and humidity are varied, and the flow rates for the tests are not those actually encountered in the job. Reworking the certification program test criteria for gas/vapor respirators is necessary in order that the laboratory be capable of extrapolating test results to those that will be obtained in actual usage situations.

In the past decade there has been a large increase in the number of women in the workplace. In 1981 women accounted for 43% of the total worker population as compared to 38% in 1973 [5]. This increase in the population of working women has been due largely to economic needs. Also, most women entering the working world do so with the intent of remaining there for their working life. With this increase in the female worker population comes the threat that more women are now being exposed to toxic dusts, chemicals and other hazardous materials.

Traditionally, most occupational health data and research have been based on the working man. This holds true for respiratory protection also. It was only in 1976 when McConville et al published a report on human variability and respirator sizes [6]. This lead to the availability of more sizes in respirators, but still did not provide the quantities that were needed. Also, there is not enough evidence available to indicate that women respond to toxic materials in the same way or differently than men do. Maybe the respirator chosen adequately protects the male workers but does not provide the necessary protection required for the female workers. There is a tremendous need for research into respiratory protection and female workers.

Traditionally, testing of performance efficiency of any respirator has been done in the laboratory. Very little information has been gathered to determine the respirator's performance in the workplace and the ability to extrapolate laboratory tests to actual field performance. More research is needed to determine the effectiveness of various respirators in various workplace conditions. This work has to be done in the workplace environment. These comments also pertain to the protection factors presently assigned to different types of respirators. These protection factors have been determined in the lab. Methods must be developed to determine actual workplace-protection factors for each respirator type. These methods should be simple to perform and should be inexpensive to the employer considering the fact that they may ensure that the respirator will be used.

Face fit is a critical aspect of the respirator-wearer interface that determines the overall protection provided by the respirator. It is vital that the face fit of a respirator be determined with a certain degree of reliability and accuracy. Presently there are qualitative and quantitative methods available, each with its advantages and disadvantages (discussed in more detail in Chapter 3). Few employers use either qualitative and quantitative fit tests to aid them in their selection of proper respiratory protection. Now OSHA, and other regulatory agencies throughout the world, are attempting to mandate the use of fit tests by the employer and the employee. There is an ever-increasing need to investigate the validity of the fit testing methods that have been developed to date and there is a need to determine the correlation between qualitative and quantitative methods. Hardis et al's article published in 1983 is a start in the right direction [7].

Advances have been made over the past twenty to thirty years in the development of respiratory protection. Respirators today are more effective, more economical, more comfortable and are more widely used, but, as has been discussed, there are a number of unanswered questions and problems that must be investigated. Future research into respiratory protection must be undertaken in order that employers be able to provide the necessary respiratory protection and be confident in their ability to protect their workforce, and that the worker wear the respirator for extended periods of time as required. We have to strive for a better understanding of the wearer aspect of the wearer-respirator interface. This will allow us to establish better performance criteria which will lead to the development of better respirators that will perform under actual workplace conditions. The ultimate goal is to protect the worker from the inhalation of hazardous or potentially hazardous materials.

## REFERENCES

1.  Morgan, W.P., "Psychological Problems Associated with the Wearing of Industrial Respirators: A Review." *Am. Ind. Hyg. Assoc. J.* 44:671–676 (1983).
2.  Ryan, C., Breyesse, P.N., White, N. and Corn, M., "Critical Review of International Standards for Respiratory Protective Equipment–I. Respiratory Protective Equipment for Particulate-Laden Atmospheres." *Am. Ind. Hyg. Assoc. J.* 44:756–761 (1983).
3.  Breyesse, P.N., White, N., Ryan, C.M., and Corn, M., "Critical Review of International Standards for Respiratory Protective Equipment–II. Gas and Vapor Removal Efficiency and Fit Testing." *Am. Ind. Hyg. Assoc. J.* 44:762–767 (1983).
4.  White, N., Ryan, C.M., Breyesse, P.N., and Corn, M., "Critical Review of International Standards for Respiratory Protective Equipment–III. Practical Performance Tests." *Am. Ind. Hyg. Assoc. J.* 44:768–773 (1983).
5.  Stellman, J.M., and Stellman, S.D., "Occupational Lung Disease and Cancer Risk in Women." *Occupational Health Nursing.* 31, 40 (1983).
6.  McConville, J.T., Churchill, E., and Laubach, L.L., "Human Variability and Respirator Sizing." Contact No. HSM-99-73-15, DHEW, NISOH (1976).
7.  Hardis, K.E., Cadens, C.A., Carlson, G.J., Da Roza, R.A., and Held, B.J., "Correlation of Qualitative and Quantitative Results from Testing Respirator Fit." *Am. Ind. Hyg. Assoc. J.* 44:78–87 (1983).

# Index

ACGIH (American Conference of Governmental Industrial Hygienists), 40, 43, 146
AWSI, 68, 70, 76
Abrasives, 20
Absorption, 66, 76
Adequate instruction, 140
Adhesives, 20
Administrator, 108, 109, 115, 124
Administration, 107, 139, 140
Administrative controls, 36, 152
Adsorption, 66, 76
Aerodynamic diameter, 11
Aerosol, 9, 10, 11, 41, 147, 154
Aging, 144
Agricultural chemicals, 84
Air curtains, 146
Airline respirator, 90, 142, 148, 149
Air purifying respirators, 48, 55, 56, 69, 70, 74, 94, 97, 98, 117, 146
Air sampling, 41, 43, 142, 145
Allergic reactions, 14
Allergies, 120
Aluminosis, 17
Alveolar duct, 5, 6
Alveolar sac, 5, 6
Alveoli, 3, 5, 6, 10, 15
Ammonia, 140
Approval of respirators, 82
Area sampling, 37
Asbestos, 144, 145, 147, 148
Asbestosis, 17, 119
Asphalt paving, 20
Asthma, 120
Atmosphere supplying respirators, 48, 70, 74, 94, 97, 98, 119
Automotive, 20, 143

BS 2091, 84
BS 4275, 85
BS 4400, 85
BS 4555, 84
BS 4558, 84
BS 4667, 84
BS 6016, 85
Bakeries, 20
Banana oil, 98
Battery manufacture, 20
Beards, 149
Berylliosis, 17
Beverage manufacture, 21
Blasting abrasive, 21, 75, 90, 146
Boiler making, 21
Brake lining, 148
Breakthrough, 66
Breathing resistance, 54, 117, 152, 153
Brewing, 21, 140
Brick manufacture, 21
British Standards Institution, 82, 84, 85
Bronchi, 5, 6, 11, 13
Bronchiole, 5, 6, 11, 13
Bronchitis, 16, 17, 18, 118, 120
Bureau of mines, 82
Business machines, 21
Byssionsis, 18

Can manufacture, 21
Carbon dioxide, 140
Ceiling value, 43
Cement manufacture, 21
Charcoal filters, 143
Charcoal production, 22
Chemical cartridge respiration, 48, 58, 60, 66, 67, 82, 90, 126, 143
Chemical hazard, 1

157